ABC of
Practical Procedures

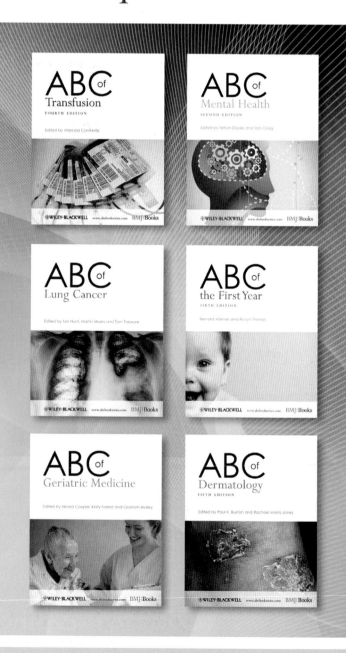

ABC of

Practical Procedures

EDITED BY

Tim Nutbeam

Specialist Trainee in Emergency Medicine
West Midlands School of Emergency Medicine
Birmingham, UK

Ron Daniels

Consultant in Anaesthesia and Critical Care
Heart of England NHS Foundation Trust
Birmingham, UK

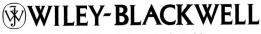 WILEY-BLACKWELL

A John Wiley & Sons, Ltd., Publication

BMJ|Books

This edition first published 2010, © 2010 by Blackwell Publishing Ltd

BMJ Books is an imprint of BMJ Publishing Group Limited, used under licence by Blackwell Publishing which was acquired by John Wiley & Sons in February 2007. Blackwell's publishing programme has been merged with Wiley's global Scientific, Technical and Medical business to form Wiley-Blackwell.

Registered office: John Wiley & Sons Ltd, The Atrium, Southern Gate, Chichester, West Sussex, PO19 8SQ, UK

Editorial offices: 9600 Garsington Road, Oxford, OX4 2DQ, UK
The Atrium, Southern Gate, Chichester, West Sussex, PO19 8SQ, UK
111 River Street, Hoboken, NJ 07030-5774, USA

For details of our global editorial offices, for customer services and for information about how to apply for permission to reuse the copyright material in this book please see our website at www.wiley.com/wiley-blackwell

The right of the author to be identified as the author of this work has been asserted in accordance with the Copyright, Designs and Patents Act 1988.

Library of Congress Cataloging-in-Publication Data

ABC of practical procedures / edited by Tim Nutbeam, Ron Daniels.
       p. ; cm. -- (ABC series)
   Includes bibliographical references and index.
   ISBN 978-1-4051-8595-0
1. Clinical medicine--Handbooks, manuals, etc I. Nutbeam, Tim. II. Daniels, Ron, MD. III. Series: ABC series (Malden, Mass.)
[DNLM: 1. Therapeutics--methods. 2. Clinical Competence. 3. Diagnostic Techniques and Procedures. 4. Inservice Training.
WB 300 A134 2010]
   RC55.A23 2010
   616--dc22

                                                                                              2009021675

ISBN: 978-1-4051-8595-0

A catalogue record for this book is available from the British Library.

Set in 9.25/12 pt Minion by Newgen Imaging Systems (P) Ltd, Chennai, India
Printed and bound in Malaysia by KHL Printing Co Sdn Bhd

1   2010

Contents

Contributors

Matt Boylan

Emergency Medicine Registrar
HEMS Doctor
Midlands Air Ambulance
DCAE Cosford, UK

Mike Byrne

Anaesthetic Registrar
Birmingham Heartlands Hospital
Bordesley Green East
Birmingham, UK

Ron Daniels

Consultant in Anaesthesia and Critical Care
Heart of England NHS Foundation Trust
Birmingham, UK

Anna Fergusson

CT2 Anaesthetics
Russells Hall Hospital
Dudley, UK

Michael Foster

Consultant Urologist
Heart of England NHS Foundation Trust
Good Hope Hospital
Birmingham, UK

Caroline Fox

Lecturer
Birmingham Women's Hospital
Birmingham, UK

Chris Hetherington

Consultant in Emergency Medicine
Worcestershire Acute Hospitals NHS Trust
Alexandra Hospital
Redditch, UK

Lucy Higgins

Academic Clinical Fellow
Maternal and Fetal Health Research Centre
University of Manchester
St Mary's Hospital
Manchester, UK

Julian Hull

Consultant Anaesthetist and Critical Care Clinical Lead
Heart of England NHS Foundation Trust
Good Hope Hospital
Birmingham, UK

Andrew King

Clinical Research Fellow
Centre for Liver Research
University of Birmingham
Birmingham, UK

Simon Laing

ST2 Emergency Medicine
City Hospital
Birmingham, UK

Lynn Lambert

Consultant in Acute Medicine
University Hospital Birmingham
Birmingham, UK

Kathryn Laver

CT2 Anaesthetics
Birmingham City Hospital
Birmingham, UK

Adam Low

CT2 Anaesthetics
University Hospital Birmingham
Birmingham, UK

Kate McCann

Paediatric Registrar
New Cross Hospital
Wolverhampton, UK

Oliver Masters

Specialist Registrar in Anaesthesia
Queen Elizabeth Hospital
Birmingham, UK

Rob Moss

ST3 Anaesthetics
Mersey Rotation
Liverpool, UK

Randeep Mullhi

Specialist Registrar in Anaesthesia
Department of Anaesthesia
Queen Elizabeth Hospital
Birmingham, UK

Anne Mutlow

Matron for Critical Care
Critical Care Unit
Heart of England NHS Foundation Trust
Good Hope Hospital
Birmingham, UK

Tim Nutbeam

Specialist Trainee in Emergency Medicine
West Midlands School of Emergency Medicine
Birmingham, UK

Ronan O'Leary

Specialist Registrar in Anaesthesia
Yorkshire Deanery
York, UK

Helen Parry

ST2 Doctor
University Hospital Birmingham
Birmingham, UK

Sharat Putta

Specialist Registrar, Liver
Queen Elizabeth Hospital
Birmingham, UK

Andrew Quinn

Consultant in Anaesthesia and Intensive Care
Department of Anaesthesia
Bradford Royal Infirmary
Bradford, UK

Nicola Sinden

Specialist Registrar in Respiratory Medicine
West Midlands Rotation
Birmingham, UK

Amy Walker

Specialist Registrar in Paediatrics
Department of Neonatology
Birmingham Women's Hospital
Birmingham, UK

Preface

This book is written as a practical guide to procedures commonly performed by healthcare professionals. It is designed to cover all the anatomy, physiology and pharmacology needed to perform a wide range of procedures competently and confidently. Each procedure is described in a detailed step-by-step manner, with supporting photographs to aid understanding. Uniquely, each chapter is written by those who perform the procedures on an everyday basis (mostly junior doctors), supported by those who supervise and teach them.

Introductory chapters introduce the fundamentals of consent, documentation, universal precautions and infection control in the context of practical procedures, and the practice of local anaesthesia and safe sedation.

The procedures themselves are divided by purpose:

Sampling: obtaining samples for laboratory analysis: blood taking and cultures, arterial blood gases, lumbar puncture and pleural tap.

Access: securing venous access: venous cannulation, insertion of a central venous catheter and specialist emergency access techniques.

Therapeutic: techniques to directly improve or stabilise a patient's clinical condition: basic and advanced airway manoeuvres, draining of ascitic fluid and insertion of chest drain.

Monitoring: procedures for intensive monitoring: urinary catheterisation, central line monitoring and arterial line insertion.

Specials: specialist procedures within emergency medicine, paediatrics and obstetrics and gynaecology.

This book is directed towards every healthcare professional who performs or assists in practical procedures throughout all healthcare environments. The syllabus for junior doctor training in the UK, including introductory specialist training, was used in the selection of the procedures.

We hope this book will prove useful as a learning tool to junior healthcare staff and as an aide memoire to more senior staff to ensure the best possible training in this practical field.

Acknowledgements

We are grateful to Anna Fergusson for compiling the Handy Hints boxes and to Simon Williams for taking many of the photographs.

Tim Nutbeam
Ron Daniels

CHAPTER 1

Introduction

Tim Nutbeam[1] and Ron Daniels[2]

[1]*West Midlands School of Emergency Medicine, Birmingham, UK*
[2]*Heart of England NHS Foundation Trust, Birmingham, UK*

OVERVIEW

By the end of this chapter you should be able to understand:
- the importance of becoming proficient at practical procedures
- the principle of 'competency'
- how to learn and maintain these skills
- the principles and purpose of a logbook.

Practical procedures

The importance of practical procedures and of performing them safely cannot be underestimated. Healthcare professionals (HCPs) will be expected to perform a wide range of practical procedures with competence and confidence. Some of these procedures will be diagnostic, some therapeutic and others life-saving. The structure of healthcare organisations dictates that even the most junior trainees will on occasion have to undertake some of the procedures described in this book without supervision.

This book contains procedures that are a part of medical, nursing and allied health curriculi throughout the world. The focus is on understanding not just the practical aspects of how to do a particular procedure but also why, when and where to do it.

Competency

Throughout healthcare education, 'competency-based training' has evolved to address gaps between theory and practice. The purpose is to demonstrate that an individual has received training and assessment in knowledge and skills relevant to all aspects of their clinical practice. Perhaps most importantly, maintaining a portfolio of competencies stimulates the trainee and their clinical supervisor to reflect on their professional development and training needs frequently to help direct future learning goals and strategies. An additional benefit may be to limit the susceptibility of practitioners, trainers and organisations to successful litigation should complications occur. Up to 50% of incidents where patients come to physical harm in hospital are due to practical procedures being inadequately

or incompetently performed. Those responsible for the training and supervision of the HCPs performing these procedures are under increasing pressure to ensure the skills required to perform these procedures are adequately taught and maintained. To do this a learning and assessment process must be demonstrated.

Becoming adept at the practical procedures expected of you within your role is a key step in achieving overall clinical competence.

A competency relates to performing a single skill or procedure, but also includes the underlying knowledge, abilities and attitudes necessary for optimal performance. In order to assess competency in a procedure it must be performed to a specific standard under specific conditions – standards and conditions this text attempts to outline. Competence also implies a minimum level of proficiency which must be attained and maintained; in the United Kingdom, case law dictates that an individual must perform a procedure to the standard which can reasonably be expected of others with a similar level of training and experience.

Learning practical procedures: attaining competency

The days of 'see one, do one, teach one' are over. Experts estimate that each new practical competency (e.g. intravenous cannulation) must be performed a minimum of 30 times to be 'learned' as a new psychomotor process; it is more difficult to estimate how frequently the process must be performed to be retained.

More complex procedures (e.g. insertion of a central venous catheter) must be performed on 50–80 occasions before an 'acceptable' level of failure/complication (5%) is reached. However, healthcare now strives to achieve an adverse event rate of fewer than 1 in 100 episodes, and in anaesthesia and blood transfusion fewer than 1 in 1000 episodes result in adverse events. A failure rate of 5%, therefore, may become unacceptable to patients in the foreseeable future.

It is impossible to generalise competency to a certain number of procedures for all individuals; the number needed to become and remain competent will vary vastly depending on the experience and dexterity of the practitioner, the procedure, how regularly it is performed, who it is performed upon and the environment in which it is performed.

There are a number of essential preconditions that a practitioner must satisfy before embarking upon a practical procedure.

ABC of Practical Procedures. Edited by T. Nutbeam and R. Daniels. © 2010
Blackwell Publishing, ISBN: 978-1-4051-8595-0.

Background knowledge

Before attempting a new procedure it is essential to gain sufficient background knowledge to attempt the procedure competently. This is not just 'how' to do a procedure but also why and when it should be done, what contraindications to it exist, the anatomy behind the procedure and its potential complications. This knowledge can be attained from discussions, teaching sessions and prereading. This book attempts to comprise the essential preprocedure reading for each of the procedures covered.

Equipment

The practitioner should attempt to familiarise themselves with the equipment used for a procedure. Equipment will vary both between hospitals and between departments within the same hospital. Familiarise yourself before you have to perform a potentially life-saving procedure; an emergency situation is not the time to have to learn the basics.

Mannequins

Mannequins are a great way to familiarise yourself with a new procedure and also maintain familiarity with a previously learnt procedure in a safe way. They are especially useful for infrequently performed, potentially dangerous procedures such as surgical chest drain insertion. Mannequins alone are not an acceptable substitute for multiple supervised procedures on 'real' patients. Other forms of substitute training include the use of animal models, which carries ethical implications, and high-fidelity simulation. This latter mode of training incorporates training in practical skills with realistic real-time scenarios, and includes elements of interprofessional working.

Patients

Patients are not there to be practised upon without knowing the experience and role of the practitioner. They should be made fully aware of your position as a trainee and the role of your trainer. A vast majority of patients will not withdraw consent: they appreciate the need for junior HCPs to learn.

Logbooks and assessment forms

It is essential to keep a logbook of the practical procedures you perform. Many professions (e.g. anaesthesia) have mandatory logbooks for all trainees provided by their governing body. A logbook shows not only the number of procedures performed but also how frequently and under what circumstances. The logbook should not contain patients' personal details, although unique identifiers (e.g. their hospital number) are permitted.

Additionally, a number of the professions now encourage regular assessment of individuals' performance in practical procedures. This may take the form of a practical mannequin-based test (ideal to test emergency situations which infrequently occur) or an assessment of how the procedure is performed for 'real'. It is essential that assessments in whatever form evaluate knowledge, skills and abilities; preferably in a multidimensional manner.

Summary

Practical procedures form an essential part of diagnosis and treatment, and may be life-saving. A healthcare professional due to undertake a procedure must be satisfied that he or she possesses the required knowledge and skills to perform it – in other words, that he or she is competent. This competence may have been assessed through informal supervision in a number of the procedures, or, increasingly, through formal 'competency-based training'.

This book provides the knowledge required to understand the reasons for performing each of the procedures described herein, together with their contraindications, the relevant anatomy and potential complications. This, together with a step-by-step guide to performing each procedure should provide the practitioner with a robust grounding to proceed to practice under supervision and ultimately competence.

CHAPTER 2

Consent and Documentation

Tim Nutbeam

West Midlands School of Emergency Medicine, Birmingham, UK

OVERVIEW

By the end of this chapter you should:
- understand the components that make up 'valid consent'
- understand the principles by which we treat patients who lack capacity
- understand the principles by which we treat children under the age of 16
- understand the importance of thorough documentation.

Introduction

In the vast majority of cases a patient must give consent in order for a procedure to be performed. The principles of valid consent are a cornerstone of all medical practice, and therefore protected by medical law. Without valid consent (or an alternative recognised by medical law) any procedure performed upon a patient is considered an assault and criminal charges may result as consequence of this.

Medical law concerning consent varies vastly from country to country – although the same principles can be found across the globe. This chapter deals primarily with the law governing patients treated in the UK.

In order for consent to be valid the following components must be present:
- capacity
- information
- voluntariness.

Capacity

'You must work on the presumption that every adult patient has the capacity to make decisions about their care, and to decide whether to agree to, or refuse, an examination, investigation or treatment'.

Consent: patients and doctors making decisions together.
GMC, June 2008

The principle of capacity is complex and variable. A patient may have the capacity to consent for a minor procedure such as phlebotomy but may lack the capacity to consent for a procedure with potentially more serious consequences such as a chest drain. Assessment of capacity is complicated and varies vastly across the globe.

In England and Wales the following two questions must be asked:
- Does the person have an impairment of, or a disturbance in the functioning of, their mind or brain?
- Does the impairment or disturbance mean that the person is unable to make a specific decision when they need to?

Or alternatively a patient lacks capacity if:
'the patient is incapable of acting on, making, communicating, understanding, or remembering decisions by reason of mental disorder or inability to communicate due to physical disorder'

Consent: patients and doctors making decisions together.
GMC, June 2008

Capacity can be seen to have four individual elements, which all must be complete in order for a patient to consent for a particular procedure.

Understanding
The patient must understand: why the procedure is being done; what the benefits and risks of the particular procedure are; what the alternatives to the procedure are; and that they have the right to refuse for the procedure to be performed.

Believing
The patient must believe the information given by the healthcare professional and understand it to be true.

Retaining
The patient must retain (and be able to recall) the information given by the healthcare professional; in non-urgent procedures giving written information may aid this process.

Weighing
The patient must weigh up the information given by the healthcare professional and make a decision. This decision is not necessarily one which the healthcare professional would have made themselves:
'This right of choice is not limited to decisions which others might regard as sensible. It exists notwithstanding that the reasons for making the choice are rational, irrational, unknown or even non-existent.'
Lord Donaldson 1992

Without all four elements of 'capacity' present the patient cannot give valid consent for a procedure to take place.

ABC of Practical Procedures. Edited by T. Nutbeam and R. Daniels. © 2010 Blackwell Publishing, ISBN: 978-1-4051-8595-0.

Box 2.1 **Mental Capacity Act 2005 – Section 1**

1 A person must be assumed to have capacity unless it is established that they lack capacity.
2 A person is not to be treated as unable to make a decision unless all practicable steps to help him do so have been taken without success.
3 A person is not to be treated as unable to make a decision merely because he makes an unwise decision.
4 An act done, or decision made, under the Act for or on behalf of a person who lacks capacity must be done, or made, in his best interests.
5 Before the act is done, or the decision is made, regard must be had to whether the purpose for which it is needed can be as effectively achieved in a way that is less restrictive of the person's rights and freedom of action.

If an adult patient lacks capacity they cannot consent for a procedure: no one may give consent for the procedure in their stead (apart from under a legally appointed Lasting Power of Attorney).

Information

The General Medical Council (UK) makes recommendations about the minimum amount of information a patient should be given in order to give valid consent for a procedure (Box 2.2). As research suggests that many patients have poor recall of oral information, written information should ideally be provided.

The information should be delivered using clear, non-technical language which the patient can understand. Consideration should be given to the use of an interpreter if there is any doubt as to the patient's ability to understand the healthcare professional due to a language barrier.

Any questions about the procedure a patient may ask must be answered in an open and honest manner.

In an emergency it may not be possible to give all the information detailed in Box 2.2; however, the patient should be aware of the purpose of the procedure, its potential side-effects and alternative treatment strategies. Any questions they have must be answered.

Voluntariness

The patient must agree to the procedure being proposed and not feel pushed or coerced into the procedure. The healthcare professional must check that the patient is in agreement for the procedure to go ahead. Particular care must be taken with patients in police custody or detained under mental health legislation.

Recording consent

If the above elements are present then a patient may consent to a procedure.

Consent to medical treatment may be oral or written, expressed or implied.

Standard consent forms are routinely used throughout medical practice and ideally should be used for the majority of medical procedures – especially those with potentially serious side-effects.

Box 2.2 **Information required for consent**

You must give patients the information they want or need about:
• the diagnosis and prognosis
• any uncertainties about the diagnosis or prognosis, including options for further investigations
• options for treating or managing the condition, including the option not to treat
• the purpose of any proposed investigation or treatment and what it will involve
• the potential benefits, risks and burdens, and the likelihood of success, for each option; this should include information, if available, about whether the benefits or risks are affected by which organisation or doctor is chosen to provide care
• whether a proposed investigation or treatment is part of a research programme or is an innovative treatment designed specifically for their benefit
• the people who will be mainly responsible for and involved in their care, what their roles are, and to what extent students may be involved
• their right to refuse to take part in teaching or research
• their right to seek a second opinion
• any bills they will have to pay
• any conflicts of interest that you, or your organisation, may have
• any treatments that you believe have greater potential benefit for the patient than those you or your organisation can offer.

Consent: patients and doctors making decisions together.
GMC, June 2008

Box 2.3 **Conditions in which written consent is recommended**

• The investigation or treatment is complex or involves significant risks.
• There may be significant consequences for the patient's employment, or social or personal life.
• Providing clinical care is not the primary purpose of the investigation or treatment.
• The treatment is part of a research programme or is an innovative treatment designed specifically for their benefit.

Consent: patients and doctors making decisions together.
GMC, June 2008

Box 2.3 covers situations when written consent is particularly recommended.

'You must use the patient's medical records or a consent form to record the key elements of your discussion with the patient. This should include the information you discussed, any specific requests by the patient, any written, visual or audio information given to the patient, and details of any decisions that were made'.

Consent: patients and doctors making decisions together.

GMC, June 2008

When consent cannot be given

When an adult patient lacks capacity to give consent and no-one with a legal power of attorney has been appointed (or cannot be contacted in an emergency situation) then a senior healthcare professional will need to decide what treatment is in the patient's best interest (Box 2.4).

The treatment or procedure should be what is:
- in the patient's best interests (taking into account the patient's past wishes and feelings)
- the minimum intervention which is required to achieve the desired purpose.

When it is reasonable and practicable to do so (i.e. in every non-emergency situation) you must consult with relevant others: family members, principal carers, etc. Specialised consent forms are used in this situation and must be signed by two senior doctors (ideally consultants) who are responsible for the patient's care.

Children and consent

The law regarding children's consent is complicated and regularly updated.

The healthcare professional should involve children as much as is practically possible in discussions about their care; this is the case even if the ultimate decision or 'consent' does not lie with the child.

In the UK and most of the developed world a young person is assessed on an individual basis on their ability to understand and weigh up options, rather than on their age. This ability to take decisions is known as 'Gillick' competence and originated from a court case regarding the prescription of oral contraceptives to young people under the age of 16.

'As a matter of Law the parental right to determine whether or not their minor child below the age of sixteen will have medical treatment terminates if and when the child achieves sufficient understanding and intelligence to understand fully what is proposed.'

Lord Scarman, 1985

If a child is judged as Gillick competent they can consent to a procedure and this decision cannot be overruled by their parents.

If a child is not Gillick competent they can neither give nor withhold consent. Those with parental responsibility need to make a decision on their behalf.

Any further detail is beyond the scope of this text. It is important to involve senior clinicians with overall responsibility for the child as early as possible in the decision-making process.

Documentation

Good medical records are essential for delivering good patient care. They are principally used to improve continuity of care and prevent medical error. They are also a vital source of information if a negligence claim is made against a healthcare professional.

The General Medical Council of the UK states:

'keep clear, accurate and legible records, reporting the relevant clinical findings, the decisions made, the information given to patients, and any drugs prescribed or other investigation or treatment; make records at the same time as the events you are recording or as soon as possible afterwards'.

With particular reference to practical procedures, as a minimum standard you should document the following.

- The time, date, who you are and where you are.
- The name of the procedure proposed.
- Consent: details of the information you discussed, any specific requests by the patient, any written, visual or audio information given to the patient, and details of any decisions that were made.
- Monitoring: document standards of monitoring whilst the procedure was being performed (e.g. ECG, SpO_2).
- Drugs administered: supplemental oxygen, sedative agents etc.
- Persons present: the name of anyone assisting or supervising the procedure (and their grade).
- Sterile precautions: include universal precautions (gloves, apron etc.) as well as additional: visor, sterile field etc.
- Sterilising agents: what was used to clean the area – chlorhexidine, alcohol wipe, normal saline etc.
- Local anaesthetic: what was used, in which dose and how it was given.
- The procedure itself: this will be specific to the procedure but will include anatomical location, and a 'step-by-step' documentation of the procedure.
- Complications: document any complications (or lack of them), including how they were resolved.
- Postprocedure management: what needs to be done next (e.g. chest X-ray for central line), period of intensive observation etc.

Medical records should be clear, objective, contemporaneous, attributable and original.

Further reading

Department of Health. (2004) *Better information, better choices, better health: putting information at the centre of health.*

Department of Health. (2001) Reference guide to consent for examination or treatment.

Gillick v West Norfolk and Wisbech AHA [1986] AC 112.

General Medical Council (GMC). (2008) *Consent: patients and doctors making decisions together.*

Mental Capacity Act (2005) Code of Practice.

Medical Protection Society. (2008) *Consent and young adults and children* (fact sheet).

MPS (2008) *Guide to consent in the UK.*

MPS (2008) *Medical Records Booklet.*

Royal College of Physicians, Patient Involvement Unit. (2006) *Explaining the risks and benefits of treatment options.* www.rcplondon.ac.uk/college/PIU/pi u_risk.asp

CHAPTER 3

Universal Precautions and Infection Control

Anne Mutlow

Critical Care Unit, Heart of England NHS Foundation Trust, Good Hope Hospital, Birmingham, UK

OVERVIEW

By the end of this chapter you will:
- understand the importance of infection control
- be able to describe the various levels of hand hygiene
- understand the term 'universal precautions'
- be able to set up a sterile field
- understand the various methods of achieving asepsis
- know what to do if a needlestick or sharps injury occurs.

Infection prevention and control procedures are processes or techniques that we can use to ensure that we safeguard the patient from infection. It is essential that these techniques are followed in all patient contact situations.

Handwashing and decontamination

Good hand hygiene by healthcare workers has been shown to be the single most important preventative measure to reduce the incidence of healthcare-associated infection. It is a simple, important action that helps prevent and control cross-infection.

Every practitioner is personally responsible for their hand hygiene, and must actively seek to promote and safeguard the interests and wellbeing of patients.

Before handwashing, rings, watches and bracelets must be removed (most hospitals will allow the wearing of a plain band wedding ring only; ensure that you are aware of local policy).

There are three levels of hand hygiene.

Level 1: Socially clean

This involves the use of liquid soap and running water to remove any visible soiling of the skin. It should be used before and after each task and every patient contact. This is sufficient to prevent cross-infection.

- Apply one shot of liquid soap to wet hands and wash using a 6- or 8-point technique (see Figure 3.1).
- Rinse in warm water.
- Dry thoroughly by patting with paper towels to prevent chafing.

Level 2: Intermediate or disinfection

An alcohol hand rub is used to kill any surface skin organisms.

The hand rub should be available at all washbasins, in all clinical areas and outside any isolation areas. In areas where wall-mounted dispensers are not practical, dispensers may be attached to trolleys or smaller dispensers may be clipped to staff uniform. Alcohol gel can be used as an alternative to soap and water (only if hands are physically clean), or to disinfect the hands before an aseptic procedure.

- Hands must be physically clean before application.
- Apply alcohol hand rub to clean hands and massage using a 6- or 8-point technique (follow manufacturer's recommendations for the amount to be used) (see Figure 3.2).
- Allow to dry before beginning your next task.

Alcohol hand gel will not kill *Clostridium difficile* spores – soap and water is necessary

---

Level 3: Surgical scrub

This involves the use of a chemical disinfection and prolonged washing to physically remove and kill surface organisms in the deeper layers of the epidermis. This should be done before any invasive or surgical procedure.

- Apply a bactericidal, detergent, surgical scrub solution to wet hands and massage in using an 8-point technique, extending the wash to include the forearms.
- Ensure the hands are positioned so as to prevent soap and water running onto and contaminating the hands from unwashed areas of the arms (high hands, low elbows technique).
- Rinse in warm water.
- Dry thoroughly by patting with sterile paper towels.
- Don sterile gown and gloves.

Figure 3.3 shows areas that are commonly missed during hand hygiene processes.

Table 3.1 shows a summary of the three techniques.

ABC of Practical Procedures. Edited by T. Nutbeam and R. Daniels. © 2010
Blackwell Publishing, ISBN: 978-1-4051-8595-0.

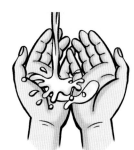
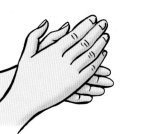
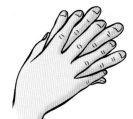

(a) Wet hands under
running water

(b) Apply soap and rub
palms together to ensure
complete coverage

(c) Spread the lather over
the backs of the hands

(d) Make sure the soap
gets in between the fingers

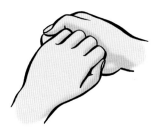
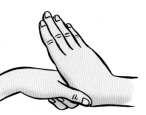
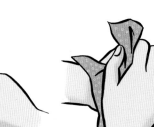

(e) Grip the fingers on
each hand

(f) Pay particular attention
to the thumbs

(g) Press fingertips into
the palm of each hand

(h) Dry thoroughly with a
clean towel

Figure 3.1 Handwashing technique. (With permission from **ECOLAB**.)

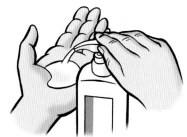
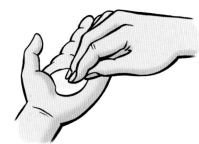
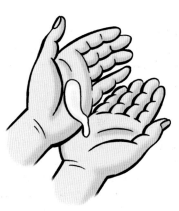

(a) Apply the gel to the palm of one hand

(b) Press fingertips of the other hand to the palm

(c) Tip the remaining alcohol from one palm
to the other

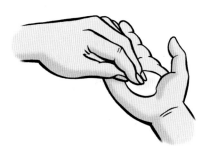
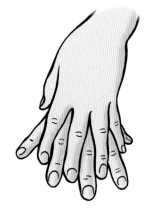
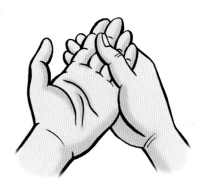

(d) Press fingertips of the other hand to the palm

(e) Quickly spread alcohol onto all
surfaces of both hands, paying particular
attention to thumbs

(f) Continue spreading the alcohol until it dries

Figure 3.2 Alcohol rub decontamination technique. (With permission from **ECOLAB**.)

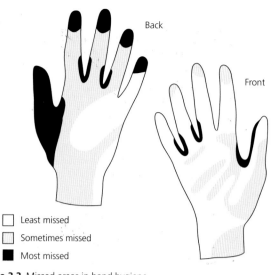

Back

Front

☐ Least missed
▦ Sometimes missed
■ Most missed

Figure 3.3 Missed areas in hand hygiene.

Table 3.1 Summary of the three levels of hand hygiene.

	Liquid soap and water	Alcohol-based handrub	Surgical scrub
	Level 1	*Level 2*	*Level 3*
Action	Removal of physical contaminants: dirt, organic matter	Killing of transient flora on physically clean hands	Disinfection and removal of transient and resident flora from hands
When	When hands are physically dirty and after using the toilet	Between patients Before applying gloves for procedures such as venepuncture, urinary catheterisation, lumbar puncture, joint aspiration, etc	Prior to surgical procedures Before applying sterile gloves to carry out a procedure where an implantable device is to be inserted such as central venous, epidural and cardiac catheters, and pacemakers

The sterile field

The sterile field is the sterile area that can be used as a work area when carrying out a sterile procedure. It is essential that this area is kept free from microorganisms and spores.

The environment

Any sterile procedures should be carried out in a clean area, free from airborne contamination. All surfaces to be used must be clean, dry, flat and stable. Any activities that will cause environmental disturbances or an increase in airborne contamination (dusting, bed-making etc.) should not be carried out immediately before an aseptic procedure. Curtains or fabric screens should be closed for 10 minutes to allow the airborne contaminates to settle. Ensure that the patient is aware of the need to maintain sterility during the procedure, as he/she may accidentally touch the sterile field.

Preparing your sterile field/trolley for the procedure

All sterile equipment is double wrapped. Packs containing sterile equipment must be unopened and the seals must be intact. The pack must be within the expiry date printed on the packaging.

All trolleys and surfaces must have been wiped or washed each day thoroughly with detergent solution. They should additionally be cleaned before each use using an alcohol-based disinfectant.

1 Wash your hands before handling the equipment and don a disposable apron and non-sterile gloves.
2 Touch only the outside layer of packaging – open the outer packs away from your body, and tip the contents onto your proposed work surface (trolley).
3 The outside of the inner wrapper is not part of the sterile field and may be touched with the hands. To open the pack, hold the corners of the wrapper only. Pull the corners out and down to expose the contents. Ensure that you do not reach across the opened pack or touch the contents.
4 The opened pack now becomes part of your sterile field.
5 Any additional sterile equipment can be tipped or dropped onto this sterile field, ensuring that the sterile surfaces are not touched.

The operator can now perform a surgical scrub and don sterile gown and gloves.

Some procedures require the operator to wear a surgical mask. This must be worn before the scrub to avoid contamination of the hands. Local policy should be adhered to.

When wearing a sterile gown and gloves, always keep your hands within view and above the waistline to prevent accidental decontamination.

Extending the sterile field

The sterile field can now be extended to include the area between the operator and the patient and surrounding the procedure site.

1 The skin is decontaminated using a bactericidal preparation of 2% chlorhexidine in 70% isopropyl alcohol, and allowed to dry.
2 Sterile drapes are opened by the operator, and held by the corners away from the body and any surfaces that will contaminate them.
3 Apply the drapes around the procedure site, also covering the area between the operator and the patient: leave only the decontaminated area of skin exposed.
4 Drapes are placed from the back to the front to avoid contaminating the operator's gown or gloves.
5 Gloves must be changed if they touch a non-sterile area.

Skin preparation solutions

Skin antisepsis before a percutaneous procedure

2% chlorhexidine in 70% isopropyl alcohol has been shown to provide very effective skin preparation. It has the dual benefits of rapid action and excellent residual activity, reducing subsequent colonisation.

Povidine iodine solution can be used if the patient has a history of chlorhexidine sensitivity.

Apply the skin preparation by rubbing the solution onto the skin commencing at the insertion site and working outwards. Rub for about 30 seconds and allow the solution to dry completely before beginning the procedure. An alternative approach, recommended for peripheral venous cannula insertion, is to use a 'criss-cross' approach in two directions to minimise the risk of missing areas.

Needlestick injury

Needlestick or sharps injuries are a daily risk for healthcare workers and can lead to infection with bloodborne viruses (BBVs) such as hepatitis or HIV. The risk of infection following a single sharps (percutaneous) injury varies depending on the type of BBV. The risk is approximately:

- 1 in 3 if the instrument is contaminated with hepatitis B
- 1 in 30 if the instrument is contaminated with hepatitis C
- 1 in 300 if the instrument is contaminated with HIV, though this depends on the infectivity of the source patient.

The chances of transmission are higher with hollow-bore needles compared to other types of sharp injury.

Prevention of needlestick and sharps injuries

There are a few simple rules to help reduce the incidence of injury.

- Do not disassemble needles from syringes or other devices – discard as a single unit.
- Do not resheath needles. If essential, use a resheathing device.
- Do not carry used sharps by hand or pass to another person.
- Discard sharps immediately after use into an approved sharps container (which you should take with you to the bedside).
- Ensure sharps containers are of an appropriate size and available at the points of use.
- Ensure sharps containers are closed securely when three-quarters full, and disposed of according to local policy.

Peripheral venous cannulae with a device that closes over the needle tip after it has been withdrawn from the cannula are available, and provide a safe option.

The risk of a percutaneous injury is increased during a surgical procedure when suture needles and scalpel blades are used. Therefore:

- use blunt suture needles where possible (not suitable for skin sutures)
- ensure that needle holders with needle tip guards are used
- use a disposable scalpel or ensure a blade removal device is used at the end of the procedure.

When taking blood samples, avoid using a needle and syringe if possible. A vacuum tube system reduces the risk of needlestick injury.

Managing accidental exposure to bloodborne viruses

Any exposure to blood or body fluids from a sharps injury, cut or bite, or from splashing into the eyes or mouth or onto broken skin, carries a risk of exposure to a BBV. All of these occurrences must be reported to, and followed up by, the occupational health team. If there is a strong suspicion of exposure to HIV, it is recommended

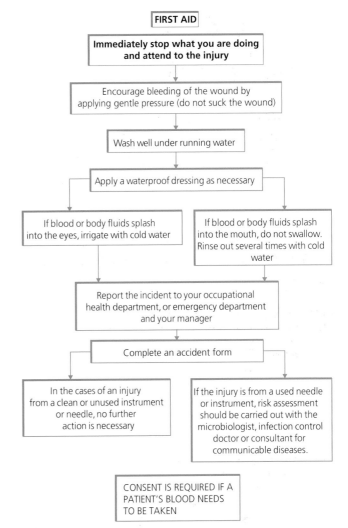

Figure 3.4 Needlestick injury protocol.

that antiretroviral post-exposure prophylaxis (PEP) is commenced. Ideally this should be started within an hour of exposure and the full course lasts 4 weeks. In situations when the treatment is delayed but the source person proves to be HIV positive, PEP can be given up to 2 weeks after the injury (though with reduced efficacy). The occupational health team will assess the circumstances and decide whether any action is necessary to reduce the risk of HIV or hepatitis.

Figure 3.4 shows what to do in the event of a needlestick/sharps injury.

Legal issues

The Human Tissue Act (HTA) 2004 was introduced following a high-profile case regarding the unethical removal and retention of organs. The act requires that virtually all organs or samples taken from humans can only be tested or stored with the explicit consent of the person from whom they were taken. Failure to obtain consent can render the offender open to a fine or imprisonment. Therefore a doctor may not test a patient for HIV or hepatitis for the benefit of an injured healthcare worker if the patient refuses the test.

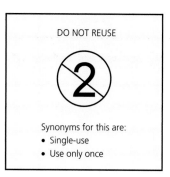

Figure 3.5 Symbol used to identify equipment that cannot be cleaned or reused.

The Mental Capacity Act (MCA) 2005 came into force on 1 October 2007. This was introduced to protect patients that lack the capacity to provide consent.

Under the MCA, all treatment decisions relating to patients over the age of 16 years who lack the capacity to consent must be necessary and made in the patient's best interests.

In the event of a needlestick injury to a healthcare worker, blood may only be taken for testing from a patient who lacks capacity or is unconscious if it is in the best interests of the patient.

Cleaning or disposing of equipment

Most equipment used in sterile procedures is disposable. Equipment that cannot be cleaned or reused can be identified by the symbol seen in Figure 3.5. Please dispose of contaminated equipment safely, and prevent injury to other healthcare workers.

Further reading

Department of Health. (2005) *Saving Lives Campaign.*

Department of Health. (2003) *Winning ways: working together to reduce healthcare associated infection in England.*

National Institute for Health and Clinical Excellence (NICE). (2003) Infection control. *NICE clinical guideline 2.* www.nice.org.uk/cg2

National Resource for Infection Control (NRIC). www.nric.org.uk.

CHAPTER 4

Local Anaesthesia and Safe Sedation

Ron Daniels

Heart of England NHS Foundation Trust, Birmingham, UK

OVERVIEW

By the end of this chapter, you should:

- be able to describe the indications for local anaesthesia and sedation
- be able to determine an appropriate agent for sedation and for local anaesthesia in an individual patient
- have an understanding of the modes of action and doses of these agents
- know the principles behind safe administration of single-agent conscious sedation
- be able to plan safe local anaesthesia including ring block
- be able to recognise and treat complications of local anaesthesia and sedation.

Introduction

Most of the practical procedures described in this book are potentially unpleasant for the patient, and a number may be painful. For some procedures, local anaesthesia and sedation will only occasionally be necessary in the adult patient (for example, peripheral venous cannulation with a small-bore cannula). For others, local anaesthesia will routinely be required (e.g. chest drain insertion). Cultural and individual factors may make sedation desirable for some patients undergoing more uncomfortable procedures.

The importance of appropriate discussion with the patient before a procedure and ongoing reassurance during it cannot be underestimated. For lengthier and more uncomfortable procedures, it is good practice to have a colleague available to hold the patient's hand and provide reassurance. Managing the patient's expectations of the procedure, being frank about the severity and duration of any likely discomfort, and explaining the reasons for performing it can minimise or negate any requirement for sedation and analgesia.

A practitioner must ensure that sedation is never administered to a patient simply to reduce the need for this basic communication. Whilst it is undoubtedly easier to practice without continually

reassuring to the patient, it is at best unsatisfactory and at worst an assault.

This chapter covers aspects of local anaesthesia and sedation relevant to the practical procedures described in this book. Specific agents in common use are described: this is not intended to be an exhaustive list. You should identify the policies and practices in use in your organisation, and familiarise yourself with which drugs and agents are available and where.

Local anaesthesia

Definition

Local anaesthesia is defined by a loss of sensation in the immediate area of the body where the agent has been administered. Effective local anaesthesia requires the blocking of transmission of pain by both Aδ (fast myelinated, 'sharp' pain) and C (slow unmyelinated, dull/throbbing pain) nerve fibres.

Local anaesthetic agents are used by anaesthetists and other experienced practitioners for both peripheral and central nerve blocks, examples being femoral nerve block and spinal (subarachnoid) block, respectively. Less commonly now, regional intravenous blockade (Biers' block) of limbs may be performed. These are specialist techniques outside the scope of this book. This chapter introduces some commonly used local anaesthetic agents, and describes their safe use in local infiltration and in performing a digital ring block.

Local anaesthetic agents

There are two principal groups of local anaesthetics – the esters (such as cocaine) and the more commonly used amides (lidocaine, bupivacaine, prilocaine). Agents differ in their potency, time to onset and duration of action according to physical properties including their lipid solubility, tendency toward protein binding and pKa (the pH at which equal proportions of ionised and non-ionised drug are present).

Local anaesthetics work by diffusing across the myelin sheath or neuron membrane in their non-ionised form. More lipid-soluble agents are more potent because more of the drug can cross into the neurone. Local anaesthetics then ionise inside the neurone, to block sodium channels from the inside (Figure 4.1). The rapidity of this process, and thus the onset of action, is determined by their pKa. The closer the pKa to physiological pH, the faster the onset. More highly protein-bound drugs will bind more strongly and have

ABC of Practical Procedures. Edited by T. Nutbeam and R. Daniels. © 2010 Blackwell Publishing, ISBN: 978-1-4051-8595-0.

a longer duration of action. The properties of the commonly used agents are listed in Table 4.1.

Most amide local anaesthetics cause local vasodilatation. Cocaine vasoconstricts, and is used in nasal surgery for analgesia and to reduce blood loss.

In the United Kingdom, the most commonly used agents are lidocaine, which has a relatively fast onset and brief duration of action; and bupivacaine and its derivative levobupivacaine, which have a slightly slower onset and longer duration.

Infected tissues are acidic, such that local anaesthetics will tend to be ionised and cross nerve membranes more slowly, and are therefore less effective.

Additives

Local anaesthetics are cleared from the site of action in the bloodstream. In more vascular areas, the duration of action of a given

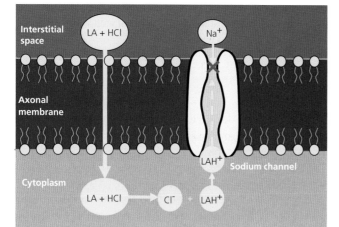

Figure 4.1 Local anaesthetics are weak bases and usually prepared as hydrochlorides (LA + HCl). At the pH of the interstitial space (7.4) they exist largely in this unionised form, which can cross the lipophilic axonal membrane with ease. Once in the cytoplasm (pH around 7.1), equilibrium shifts in favour of the ionised form (LAH$^+$, and Cl$^-$). The ionised LAH$^+$ blocks voltage-gated sodium channels from inside the cell, preventing the transmission of an action potential and thus blocking the nerve.

agent will therefore be shorter. Vasopressors, such as epinephrine and felypressin, are commercially added to some preparations to prolong the duration of action. Because systemic absorption is reduced, this may also increase the maximum safe dose of local anaesthetic for a given patient (Table 4.1). Vasoconstrictors should be avoided in the extremities, particularly the digits and the penis, because of the risk of ischaemia.

Side-effects and treatment of toxicity

At high dose, all local anaesthetics cause central nervous system (CNS) and cardiovascular effects. The CNS effects are initially excitatory, with depression occurring at higher plasma concentrations.

Initial effects include light-headedness or dizziness, and numbness or tingling around the mouth. As the plasma concentration rises, confusion, drowsiness and hypotension may ensue. With severe toxicity, convulsions, coma, respiratory arrest and cardiovascular collapse may develop. It is important to remember that, while toxicity is a spectrum, inadvertent intravenous administration can cause a patient to rapidly deterioriate to cardiorespiratory arrest.

Treatment of local anaesthetic toxicity is largely supportive, along an ABCDE format. Anticonvulsant drugs (benzodiazepines), and urgent critical care assistance for airway and ventilatory support may be required. Recently, lipid emulsions such as Intralipid® have been advocated (seek specialist advice). These lipid emulsions are of particular potential benefit in bupivacaine toxicity resulting in cardiac compromise.

Prilocaine may cause methaemoglobinaemia, which should be considered for treatment with methylene blue. Cocaine may occasionally cause coronary artery spasm and acute myocardial ischaemia. Expert help should be sought immediately if either of these rare complications are suspected.

Safe use of local anaesthetics

Naturally, a history of adverse reaction to local anaesthetic agents should be sought.

Four things are crucial:

1 to have secure intravenous access
2 to know the maximum safe dose of the agent you are using

Table 4.1 Properties of commonly used local anaesthetic agents.

Local anaesthetic	pKa	Onset	Protein binding (%)	Duration	Maximum dose (per kg ideal body weight)
Lidocaine	7.9	Rapid	64	Intermediate	4 mg/kg (7 mg/kg with epinephrine)
Bupivacaine	8.1	Intermediate	96	Long	2 mg/kg (3 mg/kg with epinephrine)
Prilocaine	7.9	Rapid	55	Intermediate	6 mg/kg (9 mg/kg with epinephrine/octapressin)
Ropivacaine: less cardiotoxic, slightly less potent than bupivacaine	8.1	Intermediate	95	Long	3 mg/kg
Levobupivacaine (s-enantiomer of bupivacaine): less cardiotoxic, ? reduced motor block	8.1	Intermediate	97	Long	3 mg/kg
Cocaine (ester): causes vasoconstriction, topical only (eyes/mucous membranes)	8.7	Slow	98	Long	3 mg/kg

3 to take steps to avoid intravascular injection

4 to seek effects of accidental intravascular injection by continually asking the patient for symptoms of early toxicity during injection.

The agent and concentration should be chosen according to the proposed site of injection, volume of solution likely to be required, and the duration of anaesthesia required. Maximum safe doses for the commonly used agents are given in Table 4.1. An example of a maximum safe dose calculation is given in Box 4.1.

Step-by-step guide: local anaesthetic infiltration

- **Give a full explanation to the patient in appropriate terms and ensure they consent to the procedure.**
- **Set up your trolley (Box 4.2).**
- **Prepare your trolley as a sterile field. Wear a plastic disposable apron and non-sterile gloves, and take alcohol hand rub with you.**

1 Ensure that the patient has no history of adverse reaction to local anaesthetic.

2 Calculate and do not exceed the maximum safe dose of your chosen agent.

3 Position the patient comfortably, with the area to be infiltrated on a secure surface.

4 Ensure that the field is adequately lit, adopt universal precautions, and set a sterile field.

5 Adequately clean the skin with an appropriate antiseptic solution (e.g. 2% chlorhexidine in 70% alcohol) and allow to dry.

6 Using a 25G (orange) or 23G (blue) needle, enter the skin at an angle of approximately 45°.

7 As soon as the needle is subcutaneous, ensure that blood cannot be aspirated. Without moving the needle, push on the plunger to infiltrate with approximately 0.5–2 mL of local anaesthetic.

8 Ask the patient if they have any tingling or numbness around the mouth, or are feeling light-headed or dizzy.

9 Advance the needle subcutaneously, avoiding superficial veins, until the tip is at the edge of the wheal just created.

10 Aspirate once more before injecting further solution.

11 Repeat steps 7–10 until the skin area is fully infiltrated, or the maximum safe dose has been reached.

12 If deeper anaesthesia is required (for example for chest drain insertion), now insert the needle into deeper tissues through the subcutaneous wheal and repeat steps 7–11 until infiltration is complete.

13 Document the agent, concentration and volume used and any complications. Allow time for the local anaesthetic to work before attempting further procedures.

14 If toxicity is suspected at any time, discontinue injection and assess using an ABCDE approach.

Step-by-step guide: digital ring block

Set up your trolley and perform steps 1–5 as for subcutaneous infiltration. There are four digital nerves per digit, one on each side toward the flexor aspect and one on each side toward the extensor

---

Box 4.1 **Example of a maximum safe dose calculation**

A 75-kg man requires infiltration anaesthesia to suture a clean laceration to the forearm.

Option 1

Bupivacaine is chosen as the agent to provide prolonged post-procedure anaesthesia. Maximum safe dose of plain bupivacaine:

- 2 mg/kg × 75 kg = 150 mg
- 0.5% bupivacaine contains 0.5 g (500 mg) of drug per 100 mL. Therefore a 10-mL ampoule of 0.5% bupivacaine contains 50 mg. *Maximum safe volume of 0.5% bupivacaine = 30 mL*

Option 2

Lidocaine is chosen to provide a quick onset of action. Maximum safe dose of plain lidocaine:

- 4 mg/kg × 75kg = 300 mg
- 1% lidocaine contains 1 g (1000 mg) of drug per 100 mL. Therefore a 10-mL ampoule of 1% lidocaine contains 100 mg. *Maximum safe volume of 1% lidocaine = 30 mL*

Box 4.2 **Equipment for local anaesthesia**

- Cleaning solution (2% chlorhexidine in 70% isopropyl alcohol recommended)
- 10-mL syringe
- Green (21G) needle for drawing up local anaesthetic from ampoule
- Orange (25G) or blue (23G) needle for infiltration
- Second 21G needle if deeper infiltration will be required
- Swabs

---

aspect (Figure 4.2). 1% lidocaine is a suitable choice of agent and will provide anaesthesia for 1–2 hours.

6 Using a 25G (orange) needle, enter the dorsal aspect of the web space, close to the phalanx on one side.

7 Advance until the tip of the needle is just above the palmar aspect of the web space.

8 Aspirate to ensure the absence of blood, then inject 1–2 mL of solution to block the palmar (volar) nerve.

9 Withdraw the needle until just under the dorsal skin.

10 Aspirate to ensure the absence of blood, then inject a further 1 mL of solution to block the dorsal nerve.

11 Ask the patient if they have any tingling or numbness around the mouth, or are feeling light-headed or dizzy.

12 Repeat steps 6–11 for the opposite side of the digit.

13 Document the procedure in the notes.

Topical local anaesthesia

Two topical local anaesthetic agents are in common use: EMLA® and Ametop®. EMLA (eutectic mixture of local anaesthetics) contains 2.5% lidocaine and 2.5% prilocaine; Ametop contains 4% tetracaine. Some systemic absorption may occur with these agents, and maximum safe doses should be observed.

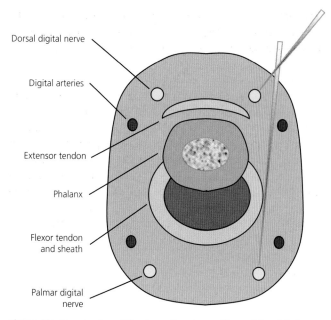

Dorsal digital nerve

Digital arteries

Extensor tendon

Phalanx

Flexor tendon
and sheath

Palmar digital
nerve

Figure 4.2 Cross-section of the finger showing positions of the digital
arteries and nerves with needle entry positions.

Each must be applied before the anticipated procedure (30 minutes
for Ametop, 60 minutes for EMLA) and covered with a waterproof,
occlusive dressing.

There is some evidence that Ametop provides slightly superior
topical anaesthesia compared with EMLA, and that it causes less
vasoconstriction which may make cannulation easier. Conversely,
skin reactions are marginally more common with Ametop.

Safe sedation

Definition
Sedation involves the use of one or more drugs to depress the CNS
to allow procedures to be carried out with minimal distress and
discomfort to the patient. It differs from general anaesthesia in that
the patient must remain conscious and in verbal contact with the
practitioner throughout the procedure.

Best practice uses a single therapeutic agent to achieve the desired
level of sedation. All drugs in common use (opiates, benzodiazepines
and others) depress the respiratory and cardiovascular systems in
addition to the CNS. These effects are compounded and become less
predictable when multiple agents are used. If analgesia using opiates
is necessary, this should be established first and time allowed for the
drug to reach its peak effect before the hypnotic agent is added.

Who can perform sedation?
Sedative drugs may be administered by a suitably qualified healthcare professional. In practice this will be a doctor, a nurse acting in
line with a Patient Group Directive, or an allied health professional
such as an Anaesthetic Practitioner. Whoever administers sedation
must be fully aware of the dose, side-effects, pharmacology and
interactions of the agent they are using.

The individual providing sedation must be adequately trained to
provide airway support and supplemental oxygen therapy, to administer bag-valve-mask ventilation and to support the cardiovascular

system up to and including external cardiac massage. The Advanced
Life Support (ALS) course provides adequate evidence of these
skills, albeit in a simulated environment. Those providing sedation
regularly should spend time with an experienced anaesthetist in
the operating theatre to hone and maintain their airway skills. Any
sedationist should be prepared to demonstrate their experience,
training and assessment in the field.

A competent individual must monitor and record the patient's
observations throughout the procedure. This may be the person
administering the sedation or the task may be delegated. If the
sedationist monitors the patient, then a second practitioner must
perform the procedure. If the task is delegated, and this individual
does not possess ALS skills, then the practitioner performing the
procedure must be prepared to abandon it immediately if complications arise from the sedation.

In other words, two qualified people are needed to safely sedate a
patient and perform a procedure.

Equipment and monitoring
Facilities should be available to administer oxygen therapy, nasally
and by face mask, from the time of onset of the sedation until the
patient is fully awake. All patient trolleys used must be capable
of being tipped 'head down', and suction should be immediately
available.

A resuscitation trolley and airway equipment – to include
oropharyngeal/nasopharyngeal airways and a means of achieving
endotracheal intubation – must be present in all areas from induc-
tion through to recovery. Emergency drugs, including antagonists
to the agents used (e.g, naloxone) should be immediately available.

An absolute minimum standard of monitoring is the continuous
presence of a trained individual, with continuous pulse oximetry
recording and verbal communication with the patient. Blood pressure and ECG recording may be advisable in lengthier procedures
or the patient with comorbidity. During recovery, a sedation score
system may be useful.

Agents in common use
Most sedation for practical procedures will be administered by
the intravenous route. If time allows, oral benzodiazepines may
be used, although at least an hour is normally required to achieve
sedation. Two classes of drug are in common use intravenously:
benzodiazepines (cause sedation, anxiolysis and amnesia), and
the anaesthetic drugs propofol (sedation) and ketamine (sedation and analgesia). Opioids (analgesia and mild hypnosis) and
Entonox® (nitrous oxide/oxygen – analgesia and euphoria) will
also be discussed briefly.

Benzodiazepines
This group of drugs, including midazolam, diazepam and loraze-
pam, act on GABAα (γ-amino butyric acid, α subgroup) receptors in the brain (Figure 4.3) by binding to specific benzodiazepine
binding sites on these larger receptors. There are two main types of
GABA receptor: α1 GABA receptors confer sedation, while the α2
subgroup cause anxiolysis. Both effects are beneficial in this instance.
Some patients will experience anterograde amnesia following the
administration of benzodiazepines, which may be unpleasant.

The sedative and anxiolytic effects of these drugs are normally apparent at a much lower dose than that needed to cause respiratory and cardiovascular depression; in comparison to propofol, they have a wider margin of safety in this respect.

Each agent has slightly differing properties, in terms of half-life, dose range, metabolites and physicochemical properties. The clinical properties are summarised for the agents in common use in Table 4.2. Arguably the most appropriate agent to use as first choice is midazolam, due to its relatively short half-life. It is also water-soluble and therefore less painful to administer intravenously than diazepam.

Most benzodiazepines have active metabolites, frequently with longer half-lives than the parent drug. For this reason, this group of drugs should only be used for sedation in the short term in normal circumstances.

Benzodiazepines are Class C controlled drugs.

Side-effects

All benzodiazepines have the potential to cause respiratory and cardiovascular system depression. Prolonged confusion and ataxia may be problematic, particularly with longer-acting agents such as diazepam. Patients may occasionally develop paradoxical excitement and aggression. Dependence and idiosyncratic reactions can occur, but are rare in the context of single-event sedation.

Antagonist

Flumazenil is a competitive inhibitor at the benzodiazepine binding site. It is available in 5-mL ampoules containing 500 microgrammes (µg) of drug. A dose of 200 µg should be administered over 15 seconds in suspected benzodiazepine overdose, with supplementary boluses of 100 µg if the patient fails to respond. It should be remembered that flumazenil has a short half-life compared with most benzodiazepines; the patient should be continually monitored for recurring sedation and the practitioner prepared to give additional doses.

NB Flumazenil is *not* suitable for administration to reverse purposeful patient-led overdose of benzodiazepine-based medication.

Anaesthetic agents

Propofol

Propofol is a drug commonly used to induce anaesthesia and to maintain sedation on critical care units. It has a narrower window of safety than benzodiazepines in that it causes respiratory depression and hypotension at doses only marginally greater than those causing sedation. It should therefore only be administered by those expert in providing airway, ventilatory and cardiovascular support.

Despite this, in experienced hands, propofol has a number of advantages over benzodiazepines. It is less likely to cause residual sedation, since it has a short duration of action and no active metabolites. Similarly, it does not accumulate to a great extent with repeated doses. Amnesia does not occur at subhypnotic doses.

Dose

Propofol is available in 1% (10 mg/mL) and 2% strengths. It is a white emulsion, formulated with egg protein and soybean oil, or in synthetic lipid suspension. An initial appropriate bolus for an average adult to achieve conscious sedation is 30–50 mg (3–5 mL of 1%), with further 10-mg boluses to achieve and maintain the desired effect (see Figure 4.4). This should be reduced in the very elderly.

Side-effects

Propofol causes respiratory depression and hypotension commonly, and may cause bradycardia. It may precipitate hiccups and

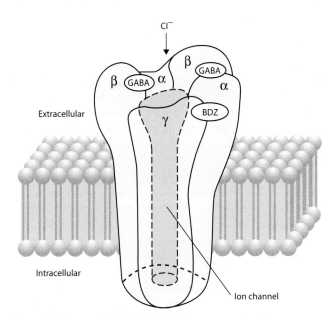

Figure 4.3 Diagram of the 5-subunit GABAα receptor, showing benzodiazepine-specific binding site (BDZ).

Table 4.2 Clinical properties of intravenous benzodiazepines used in conscious sedation.

Agent	Suggested initial IV dose	Suggested 'top-up' dose	Time to peak effect	Duration	Amnesia	Active metabolites?	Comments
Midazolam	1–2 mg	0.5–1 mg Wait 2 min	1–5 min	15–60 min	+++	None	Water soluble (at pH<4), less pain on injection
Diazepam	2.5–5 mg	1–2.5 mg Wait 5 min	2–10 min	30–90 min	+	Nordiazepam Temazepam Oxazepam	Pain on injection. Diazemuls (emulsion in lipid) less painful
Lorazepam	0.5–2 mg	0.25–1 mg Wait 15 min	10–20 min	2–6 h	++	None	Dilute before injection to reduce irritation

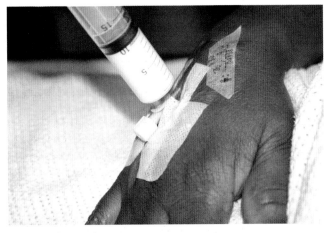

Figure 4.4 Propofol infused into peripheral cannula.

transient 'jerky' limb movements. The most common side-effect is of pain on injection, which can be reduced by adding 1 mL of 0.5% lidocaine to a 20-mL syringe.

There is no antagonist to propofol, but the clinical duration of action is brief – of the order of 20 minutes.

Ketamine

Ketamine and its active metabolite norketamine are non-competitive antagonists of the N-methyl-D-aspartate (NMDA) receptor, normally acted upon by the excitatory neurotransmitter glutamate. Ketamine has potent analgesic effects in addition to sedative and, in high dose, hypnotic effects. Its use is limited by emergence phenomena in adults including vivid hallucinations and nightmares.

Ketamine has a relatively wide therapeutic window, causing less hypotension (in fact it may cause hypertension and tachycardia) than other sedatives. It may be a suitable choice of agent in remote areas, particularly in children and the very elderly and in trauma and burns patients.

Since January 2006, ketamine has been a Class C controlled drug.

Dose

Ketamine is available in three strengths: 10 mg/mL, 50 mg/mL and 100 mg/mL. This wide range of strength demands vigilance. It is good practice to dilute any strength to 10 mg/mL for use in sedation. A suitable initial dose is 25–70 mg (or 0.5–1 mg/kg), with further doses of 15–35 mg (or 0.25–0.5 mg/kg) as required. The clinically effective duration of action is around 10–20 minutes.

Side-effects

As stated above, emergence phenomena are the most troublesome side-effect. Loss of airway is rare, and tachycardia and hypertension may result. Caution should be exercised in patients with potentially raised intracranial or intraocular pressures.

There is no antagonist to ketamine.

Opioid analgesics

These agents are used where an intervention is expected to cause moderate to severe pain. With the appropriate use of local anaesthesia, reassurance and sedation they should not be indicated for any of the procedures described in this book.

Table 4.3 Patient factors indicating the need for expert assistance.

Anatomy
Short neck
Morbid obesity, especially central
Receding jaw
Macroglossia
Facial or airway trauma
Inhalational injury to airway or oropharynx

Physiology
Daily symptoms from:
   pulmonary disease
   cardiovascular disease
   cerebrovascular disease
Hiatus hernia (symptomatic)
Obstructive sleep apnoea
Poorly controlled hypertension
Hepatic or renal failure (delayed excretion)

General
Full stomach (risk of aspiration; delay procedure if possible for 2 hours
   following clear fluids and 6 hours following food)
Previous hypersensitivity to sedative/anaesthetic agents
Nauseated or vomiting

If a practical procedure is to be performed for a patient already in pain (for example, a central venous catheter for a trauma patient), then analgesia should be addressed first. Opiates and any adjuncts should be administered to satisfactorily control the pain before any attempt at sedation. Morphine remains the most appropriate and effective opioid analgesic for the vast majority of situations, and should be titrated intravenously in the acute setting.

Entonox®

This mixture of 50% nitrous oxide and 50% oxygen can provide moderate analgesia of very brief duration for some procedures. Particular applications include labour, changes of dressings and manipulations of fractures. Benefit may be derived for some other practical procedures. Apart from the very brief duration of action, use is limited by euphoria and nausea.

Step-by-step guide: safe sedation

1 Assess the patient for any risk factors that may indicate the need for the presence of an experienced anaesthetist (Table 4.3).
2 Ensure that the patient has given their informed consent to both the procedure and the sedation.
3 Ensure that all equipment including monitoring and emergency equipment, and all drugs including emergency drugs, are checked and immediately to hand. Clarify lines of communication should complications occur (e.g. obtain contact details for on-call anaesthetist).
4 Identify the individual responsible for monitoring and recording observations, not the person administering sedation.
5 Wear non-sterile gloves and a disposable plastic apron, and consider personal protective equipment.
6 Establish and secure a peripheral venous cannula (Chapter 10).
7 Prepare the agent to be used. If not prediluted, dilute to a suitable volume (10–20 mL) to allow titration of dose, according to manufacturer's instructions.

8 Administer supplemental oxygen to the patient. Nasal cannulae with a flow rate of 2–4 L/min are suitable, but will only provide inspired oxygen levels of 24–35%.

9 Attach monitoring (minimum: continual pulse oximetry).

10 Administer an increment of sedation according to the guidelines above. Typically this will be 2–4 mL of the agent.

11 Assess for response after 2–3 minutes. The patient should be comfortable and able to talk, but calm and slightly obtunded. If the patient remains anxious or is wide awake, consider a further dose of ¼ to ½ the original bolus. Reassess and repeat again if necessary.

12 Monitor continuously by verbal communication, clinical signs and pulse oximetry (minimum).

13 Follow emergency protocols should the patient's airway be compromised or should they become unconscious.

14 If the patient becomes agitated or distressed during the procedure, give a further dose of ¼ to ½ the original bolus. Reassess and repeat again if necessary.

15 Discontinue continuous monitoring only once the patient is fully awake and all observations are satisfactory.

16 Document the agent(s) used and any complications, and ensure that the observations are recorded accurately.

Handy hints/troubleshooting

- A high standard of monitoring is essential – continuous heart rate and oxygen saturations, and intermittent non-invasive blood pressure are recommended.
- Never underestimate the potential dangers of sedation – always have a back-up plan.
- Be aware of respiratory or cardiac depression once a painful stimulus has been removed: this may be apparent after successful joint reduction.

Further reading

British National Formulary

Rosenberg PH. (2000) *Local and Regional Anaesthesia*, Wiley-Blackwell, Oxford.

UK Academy of Medical Royal Colleges and Their Faculties. (2001) *Implementing and Ensuring Safe Sedation Practice for Healthcare Procedures in Adults*. www.rcoa.ac.uk/docs/safesedationpractice.pdf

Watts J. (2008) *Safe Sedation for all Practitioners: A Practical Guide*. Radcliffe Publishing, Oxford.

Whitwam JG, McCloy RF, eds. (1998) *Principles and Practice of Safe Sedation*, 2nd edn. Blackwell Science, Oxford.

CHAPTER 5

Sampling: Blood-Taking and Cultures

Helen Parry and Lynn Lambert

University Hospital Birmingham, Birmingham, UK

OVERVIEW

By the end of this chapter you should be able to:
- understand the indications and contraindications for phlebotomy
- identify and understand the relevant anatomy
- be aware of different types of blood sampling devices
- describe the procedure of blood sampling
- appreciate when to take samples for blood culture
- use a blood culture sampling technique that minimises the risk of contamination.

Phlebotomy

Indications

- Profile testing, e.g. urea, electrolytes, liver function testing.
- Investigation of specific diseases, e.g. cortisol in Cushing's syndrome.
- Monitoring of hormones, therapeutic drugs and tumour markers.
- Toxicology, e.g. paracetamol levels.
- Venesection for therapeutic management of polycythaemia rubra vera.
- Sampling according to research protocols (ensure that you have consent).

Contraindications

- Infection at the site of access, e.g. cellulitis.
- Bleeding tendencies (relative contraindication), e.g. on warfarin
- Thrombophlebitis.
- Taking sample from 'drip arm' (stop infusion and wait for at least 2 minutes before sampling).

Points of access

- Antecubital fossa (this is the most commonly used site and contains the basilic, cephalic and median cubital veins).
- Forearm, hand and digital veins (these can often be accessed using a butterfly needle).
- Femoral vein.

Landmarks and anatomy

Antecubital fossa

The antecubital fossa contains important vasculature for venepuncture. With the arm in the anatomical position and flexed, the biceps tendon is easily palpated and is located slightly medially within the fossa. Medially is the basilic vein and this divides to produce the median cubital vein (see Figure 5.1). The median cubital

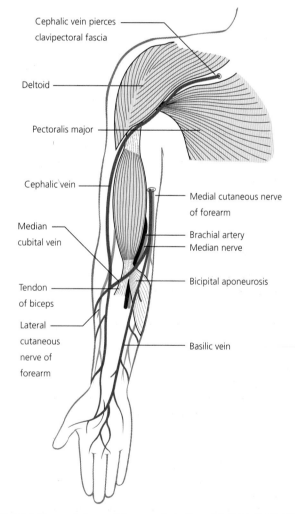

Figure 5.1 Venous drainage of the upper limb. (From Faiz O, Moffat D. (2006) *Anatomy at a Glance*, 2nd edn. Blackwell Publishing, Oxford, with permission.)

ABC of Practical Procedures. Edited by T. Nutbeam and R. Daniels. © 2010 Blackwell Publishing, ISBN: 978-1-4051-8595-0.

Table 5.1 A summary of blood collection bottles (adapted from www. vacuette.com).

Bottle lid colour	Tube contents	Tests
Purple	EDTA (ethylenediamine-tetraacetic acid)	Full blood count, ESR, malaria screen, tacrolimus, cyclosporin, HbA1c, PCR analysis, cross-match and group and save
Gold	Clotting accelerator and separation gel	Biochemistry testing, tumour markers, endocrine testing
Light blue	Trisodium citrate	Coagulation testing
Red	Clotting accelerator	Serology, vancomycin, immunology, insulin, B12, folate
Grey	Sodium fluoride/potassium oxalate	Glucose
Green	Lithium heparin	Ammonia
Royal blue	Sodium heparin	Trace elements

vein combines with the cephalic vein (located medially in the antecubital fossa.) and is often used for venepuncture.

Collection

There are different types of collection bottle depending on the test being performed. As a rule of thumb, anything for haematological investigation, group and save or DNA analysis such as PCR amplification requires blood collection in an EDTA (ethylenediaminetetraacetic acid) collection tube. This tube usually has a purple lid. Biochemical investigations are collected in tubes containing a clotting accelerator and separation gel. These are usually gold or yellow. Clotting investigations require trisodium citrate tubes which are usually light blue in colour. Table 5.1 is a guide for blood bottles in the UK. Check local guidelines for further information.

Samples should be delivered to the laboratory as soon as taken and always the same day.

Equipment: methods for blood collection

There are several means by which a phlebotomist may obtain blood The pros and cons of each can be found in Box 5.1.

Box 5.1 **Pros and cons of the different equipment used in phlebotomy**

Pros
- A Vacutainer™ system is safest.
- A needle and syringe or use of a butterfly demonstrates a flashback to confirm the needle has entered the vein.

Cons
- A multipurpose needle with a tube holder does not allow for a flashback. Therefore, until a Vacutainer™ tube is loaded onto the tube holder it is unclear if the vein has been successfully punctured.
- When using a Vacutainer™ system, the loading of different blood collection tubes whilst keeping the needle still within the vein requires some dexterity and practice.

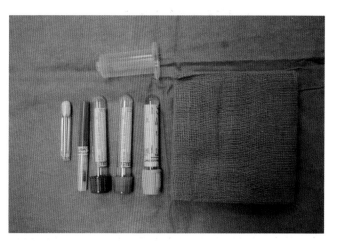

Figure 5.2 Equipment for phlebotomy.

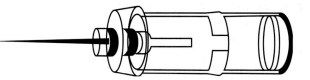

Figure 5.3 A multisampling needle and collecting tube.

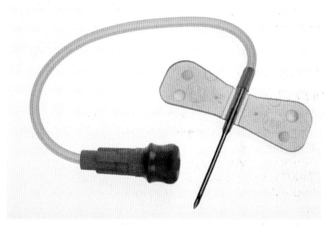

Figure 5.4 A butterfly needle.

Vacutainer™ system

One of the safest means of phlebotomy involves the use of a Vacutainer™ system. This consists of a cylindrical clear plastic collecting device, known as a tube holder, which is attached to either a multisampling needle (Figure 5.3) or a butterfly needle and luer adaptor (Figure 5.4). Vacutainer™ blood bottles are loaded onto the luer adaptor within the tube holder; the vacuum present causes blood to flow directly from the vein and into the bottle (Figure 5.5).

Needle and syringe

This is the traditional method for phlebotomy. It is simply a needle (normally 21G – green) attached to a syringe.

Step-by-step guide: venepuncture

Give a full explanation to the patient in simple terms and ensure they consent to the procedure. Prepare equipment (Figure 5.2)

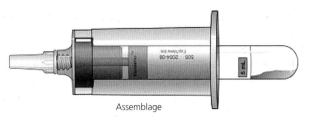

Figure 5.5 Loading of the vacutainer bottle into the tube holder.

1 Wear gloves and apron at all times.
2 Inquire whether the patient is left- or right-handed and attempt venepuncture initially in the non-dominant arm.
3 Place the tourniquet above the site of venpuncture (usually this is above the antecubital fossa) (Figure 5.6a).
4 Leave for at least 20 seconds for the veins to fill; often it is helpful at this stage if the patient makes repetitive fist actions with their hand.
5 Feel and look for access sites. Often a 'bouncy' vein that is easily palpable is far easier and generally more successful for phlebotomy rather than a visible 'thready' vein. Usually the antecubital fossa is a good starting point. If no obvious vein is found, work down the arm feeling and looking for a more suitable vein, or alternatively try the other arm.
6 Once a site of access has been decided upon, wipe the skin carefully with a antiseptic wipe (2% chlorhexidine in 70% alcohol), working in circles from the centre outwards (Figure 5.6b).
7 With the needle attached to either a Vacutainer™ system or syringe, insert the bevel upwards, passing through the skin and into the vein (Figure 5.6c).
8 Attach collecting bottles or withdraw the plunger of the syringe. Collect blood.
9 Once enough blood has been collected, loosen the tourniquet.
10 Withdraw the needle and place a cotton ball over the access site. Secure with tape.
11 Dispose of the needle appropriately in a sharps box. Never leave sharps lying around.
12 If blood has been collected in a syringe, this will now need to be transferred to bottles.
13 Label bottles with patient details. Group and save samples or cross-matching samples must always be handwritten at the patient bedside, correlating information transcribed on the bottle with the patient themselves, their hospital wrist band and the collecting form.

Complications and how to avoid them

- Infection at the puncture site. This can be minimised by cleaning the skin with an antiseptic wipe (e.g. 2% chlorhexidine/70% alcohol solution).
- Haematoma. This occurs more frequently if patients are on warfarin or steroid therapy. To avoid a haematoma, apply gentle pressure for 1–2 minutes after the procedure and release the tourniquet before removing the needle. Advise the patient to keep their arm straight.

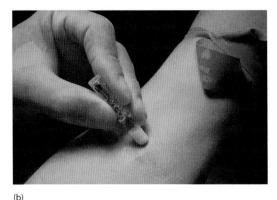

(a)

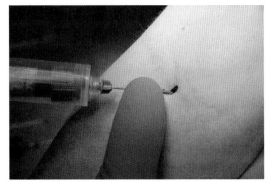

(b)

(c)

Figure 5.6 Step-by-step guide: venpuncture. (a) Apply a tourniquet to the upper arm. (b) Sterilise the skin using 2% chlorhexidine in 70% alcohol solution. (c) Attaching a collecting bottle to the Vacutainer™ system.

- Pain. This may be from the tourniquet or from venepuncture. A local anaesthetic cream may be applied to the skin to reduce the pain incurred.

Blood cultures

Indications

- To culture bacteria in cases of infection. The chances of successful culture are greatly improved if taken at the time of pyrexia.
- In the case of suspected endocarditis it is important to obtain blood from three different sites and at different times.
- If severe sepsis is present, at least one set should be drawn percutaneously and one from each indwelling vascular access device.

Step-by-step guide: blood culture

Give a full explanation to the patient in simple terms and ensure they consent to the procedure. Prepare equipment (Figure 5.7)

1 Collect culture bottles, phlebotomy equipment and antiseptic stick (Figure 5.7).
2 Identify an accessible vein.
3 Ensure the skin over the vein is sterile by using an antiseptic (2% chlorhexidine in 70% alcohol solution). Allow to dry and do

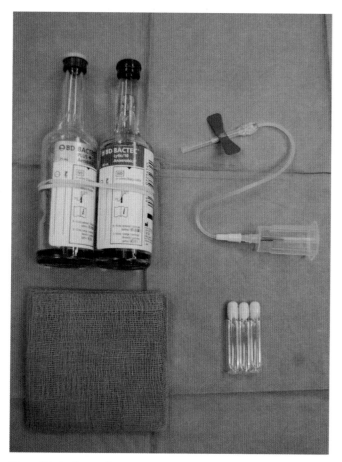

Figure 5.7 Equipment for taking cultures.

not touch the skin again after it has been cleaned (non-touch technique).

4 Clean the tops of an anaerobic and aerobic blood culture bottle using a chlorhexidine/alcohol wipe. Allow to dry fully (Figure 5.8a,b).
5 Collect at least 20 mL blood in a syringe, using a 21G (green) needle or vacutainer system (Figure 5.8c,d).
6 If using a needle and syringe, be sure to use a clean needle for each culture bottle and place at least 10 mL blood in each bottle.
7 Label fully with clinical details, antibiotics currently being administered to the patient and the time and date of the sample. Some organisations require the barcode attached to the culture bottles to be removed and either placed in the patient notes or attached to the request form. Check for local guidance.

Femoral venous access

This is used when alternative veins are unsuitable for phlebotomy, such as if the upper limbs are not accessible, if infection is present or if the patient simply has poor veins for venepuncture.

Anatomy of the femoral triangle

It is important to know the anatomy of the femoral triangle when attempting a femoral stab. It is a space found in the groin, demarcated medially by the adductor longus muscle edge (apparent by flexion, abduction and laterally rotation of the thigh), laterally by sartorius and superiorly by the inguinal ligament (this runs between the pubic tubercle and the anterior superior iliac spine). The femoral artery, nerve and vein are all found within the femoral triangle (Figure 5.9).

Sampling

1 Sampling is obtained using a 21G needle and a 20-mL syringe.
2 Palpate for the femoral artery; the femoral vein lies medial to this.
3 Wipe the skin with an antiseptic wipe (2% chlorhexidine/70% alcohol) and allow the skin to dry.
4 Insert the needle approximately 1 cm medial to the femoral artery, and at 90° to the skin, withdrawing the plunger as you advance the needle.

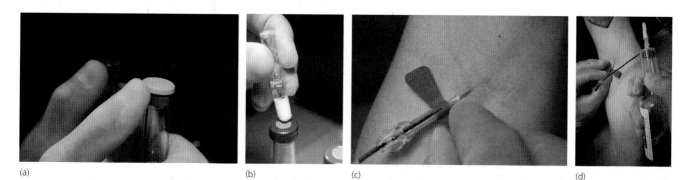

(a) (b) (c) (d)

Figure 5.8 Step-by-step guide: blood cultures. (a) Removing the tops of culture bottles. (b) Cleaning the tops of blood culture bottles using 2% chlorhexidine in 70% alcohol solution. (c) A butterfly needle inserted into a vein. (d) A blood culture sample being taken.

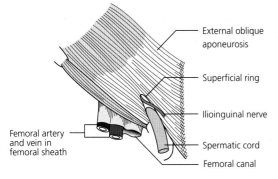

Labels in figure:
- External oblique aponeurosis
- Superficial ring
- Ilioinguinal nerve
- Femoral artery and vein in femoral sheath
- Spermatic cord
- Femoral canal

Figure 5.9 Anatomy of the femoral artery. (From Faiz O, Moffat D. (2006) *Anatomy at a Glance*, 2nd edn. Blackwell Publishing, Oxford, with permission.)

5 Once flashback is achieved, stop advancing the needle and withdraw the plunger to collect the required blood.

6 Following collection, withdraw the needle, apply pressure over the access site using cotton wool and distribute the blood into the required bottles.

Handy hints/troubleshooting

- If using the needle and syringe technique, loosen the plunger several times before taking the blood – this should avoid the plunger sticking.
- Encourage venodilation by asking the patient to repetitively clench and release his or her fist, and by gently tapping on the vein.
- Tether the skin with your spare hand to help fix the vein.
- Consider whether a cannula is also needed – if so, blood can be taken from the cannula after insertion, by using either a Vacutainer™ technique or a needle and syringe (see Chapter 10).
- Take great care when labelling cross-match and group and save samples – the smallest of errors can make the sample void. Always handwrite these samples and include all the patient's details.
- Remember femoral triangle anatomy with the acronym NAVY – from lateral to medial there is *n*erve, *a*rtery, *v*ein and then *Y*-fronts!
- Include as much clinical information on the forms as possible, especially microbiology forms.

Further reading

Bache J, Armitt C, Gadd C. (1998) *Practical Procedures in the Emergency Department*. Mosby, Oxford.

Lumley JS. (2002) Surface Anatomy. *The Anatomical Basis of Clinical Examination*, 3rd edn. Churchill Livingstone, Edinburgh.

Marbat LL, Case E. (2004) *Clinical Procedures. Blueprints*. Blackwell Publishing, Oxford.

Moore KL, Dalley AF. (1999) *Clinically Orientated Anatomy*, 4th edn. Lippincott Williams & Wilkins, Philadelphia.

CHAPTER 6

Sampling: Arterial Blood Gases

Kathryn Laver[1] and Julian Hull[2]

[1]*Birmingham City Hospital, Birmingham, UK*
[2]*Heart of England NHS Foundation Trust, Good Hope Hospital, Birmingham, UK*

OVERVIEW

By the end of this chapter you should be able to:
- understand the indications and contraindications for arterial blood gas sampling
- identify the sites used for arterial blood gas sampling
- describe different types of arterial blood gas sampling device
- describe the procedure of performing an arterial blood gas
- interpret the results of an arterial blood gas.

Introduction

Arterial blood gas (ABG) samples can be used in the assessment of critically ill or deteriorating patients, and to guide therapy in specific conditions.

Indications

All though not an exhaustive list, ABGs are useful in the following situations.

Respiratory distress (e.g. asthma, chronic obstructive pulmonary disease)
- Is the patient hypoxic (cyanosis, confusion, hallucinations)?
- Is the patient retaining carbon dioxide (drowsy, flap, headache, bounding pulse)?
- Differentiating between type I and type II respiratory failure.

Critically unwell patient (e.g. sepsis, gastrointestinal bleed, diabetic ketoacidosis, arrhythmias, impaired consciousness etc.)
- Identify and quantify acid–base disturbance.
- Quick assessment of electrolytes and haemoglobin.
- Some machines will measure lactate (a byproduct of anaerobic respiration).
- Global assessment of adequacy of fluid resuscitation (pH, lactate).

ABC of Practical Procedures. Edited by T. Nutbeam and R. Daniels. © 2010
Blackwell Publishing, ISBN: 978-1-4051-8595-0.

Box 6.1 Modified Allen's test

Occlude the patient's radial and ulnar arteries by direct pressure whilst exanguinating the hand through elevation and by asking the patient to make a fist. In an unconscious patient the hand can be squeezed so it blanches. With the hand open, release the pressure on the ulnar artery and observe the return in colour, which should occur within 6 seconds.

To guide ongoing therapy
- Assessment (e.g. of ventilation) in higher dependency environments and critical care.
- Assessment for home oxygen therapy in those with chronic respiratory and cardiac conditions.

All ABGs should be interpreted in conjunction with careful clinical assessment of the patient's condition.

Absolute contraindications
- Puncture through skin with cellulitis.
- Puncture of a vessel where there is a graft (e.g. femoral graft).
- Presence of an arteriovenous fistula in the forearm (for radial or brachial punctures).
- Underlying skeletal trauma at wrist or elbow (risk of introducing infection).
- A positive Allen test (see Box 6.1 and Figure 6.1) should prompt the physician to use an alternative site.

Relative contraindications
- Coagulation defects (e.g. liver failure, on warfarin, post thrombolysis).
- Chronic renal failure. Arterial puncture can hinder the formation of arteriovenous fistulae in the future and therefore if possible the arms should be avoided.

Arterial samples can be taken from the radial, brachial or femoral arteries. Each site has its own advantages and disadvantages (Table 6.1).

Anatomy: radial, brachial and femoral arteries

The radial artery (Figure 6.2) is relatively superficial, lying at 0.5–1 cm beneath the skin.

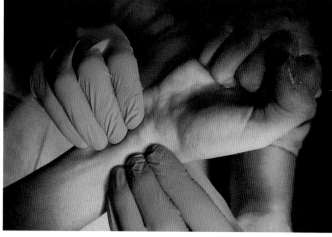
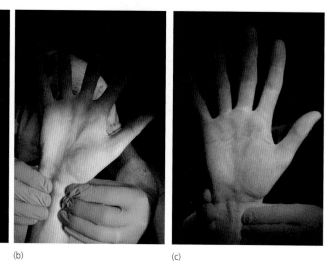

(a)

(b)   (c)

Figure 6.1 Allen's test. (a) The patient's hand is elevated and pressure applied to both the radial and ulnar arteries. (b) The patient's hand will blanch white. (c) On release of pressure over the ulnar artery the hand should re-perfuse and lose its white colouration.

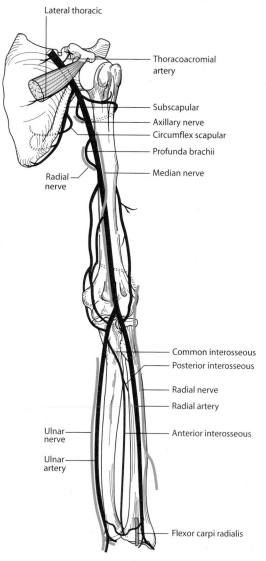

Figure 6.2 Anatomy of the radial artery. (From Faiz O, Moffat D. (2006) *Anatomy at a Glance*, 2nd edn. Blackwell Publishing, Oxford, with permission.)

Table 6.1 The points of access for arterial sample.

	Advantages	Disadvantages
Radial	Lies close to the surface Easily compressible Easy aseptic approach	End artery Pulse may be hard to feel in shut down patients or in patients with atrial fibrillation
Brachial	Can lie close to the surface Easy aseptic approach Easily compressible	End artery, quite mobile! Close proximity to the nerve
Femoral	Reliable position, good landmarks Can take other bloods at the same time Can be found in shut down patients with poor or no pulses	Dirtier' area of the body May dislodge plaque in PVD

The brachial artery (Figure 6.3) lies 0.5–1.5 cm deep, medial to the biceps tendon, with the median nerve running along its medial edge.

The femoral artery (Figure 6.4) is the deepest, at between 2–4 cm, and is found at the mid-inguinal point 2 cm below the inguinal ligament. The femoral nerve lies laterally and the vein medially.

Equipment: types of blood gas syringe

There are several types on the market and different organisations will stock different brands. The following features are present.

- Blood gas syringes contain heparin to prevent clotting of the blood (and ultimately prevent clogging of the analyser!). The heparin can be in two forms: (i) liquid; which must be expelled (leaving a thin film on the inner surface of the syringe) before procedure; or (ii) an impregnated patch in the base of the syringe.
- Some gas syringes will come in a pack with a needle, bung and cap; others will only have a cap.
- Most syringes are designed to self-fill; those that do not require traction on the plunger.

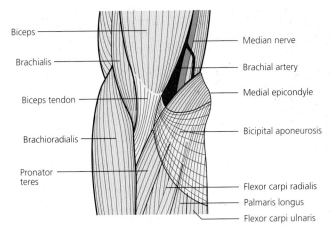

Figure 6.3 Anatomy of the brachial artery. (From Faiz O, Moffat D. (2006) *Anatomy at a Glance*, 2nd edn. Blackwell Publishing, Oxford, with permission.)

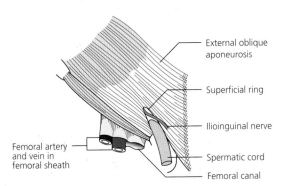

Figure 6.4 Anatomy of the femoral artery. (From Faiz O, Moffat D. (2006) *Anatomy at a Glance*, 2nd edn. Blackwell Publishing, Oxford, with permission.)

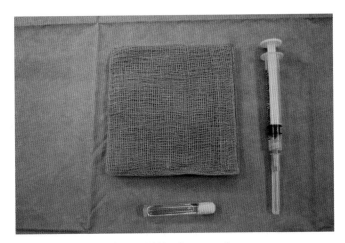

Figure 6.5 Equipment for arterial blood gas sampling.

Step-by-step guide: arterial blood gas sampling

- **Give a full explanation to the patient in simple terms and ensure that they consent to the procedure.**
- **Set up your trolley (Box 6.2; Figure 6.5).**
- **Prepare your trolley as a sterile field. Wear a plastic disposable apron and non-sterile gloves, and take alcohol hand rub with you**

Box 6.2 **Equipment for arterial blood gas sampling**

- Gloves (sterile for procedure, non-sterile for preparation)
- Skin preparation solution (2% chlorhexidine in 70% isopropyl alcohol)
- Cotton wool and tape
- Tray with sharps bin
- Arterial blood gas syringe (and needle if not provided)
- A patient label, and pen to write down their details including the inspired oxygen concentration

Attach a 21G or 23G needle to the syringe. A 21G needle is likely to be required for femoral access.

Radial

1 Conduct Allen test (Box 6.1).
2 Position the wrist; you can use a towel, pillow or bag of fluid to extend the wrist (20–30°).
3 Feel for the pulse just proximal to the traverse skin crease at the wrist (Figure 6.6a).
4 Clean the skin with antiseptic solution (2% chlorhexidine in 70% isopropyl alcohol) and put on sterile gloves (Figure 6.6b).
5 With the pulp of your fingers, assess the size, depth, direction and point of maximum pulsation.
6 Holding the syringe like a pen bevel upwards, at 45° aim at the point of maximum pulsation, in a proximal direction (Figure 6.6c).

Brachial

1 Position the arm so the medial aspect of the antecubital fossa is easily accessible.
2 Clean the skin with antiseptic solution (as above) and don sterile gloves.
3 Feel for the pulse, assessing size, depth, direction and point of maximum pulsation.
4 Holding the syringe at 45° aim at the point of maximum pulsation, in a proximal direction.

Femoral

1 Make sure the patient is lying flat.
2 Clean the skin with antiseptic solution (as above) and don sterile gloves.
3 Place fingers on the femoral pulse.
4 Aim the needle at the point of maximum pulsation, distal to your fingers at almost 90° to skin.
5 Slowly advance the needle whilst pulling back on the plunger until flashback is achieved.

All sites

1 When you enter the artery the needle should self-fill; if not keep the needle still and pull back on the plunger.
2 Collect 1–2 mL of blood (Figure 6.6d).
3 Withdraw needle and compress with cotton wool.
4 Discard needle (into sharps bin), expel the air and place the cap on the end.
5 Invert several times and take swiftly to the ABG analyser.

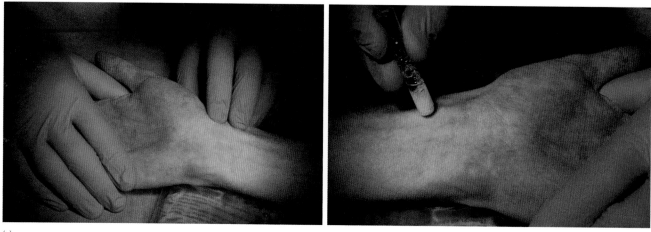

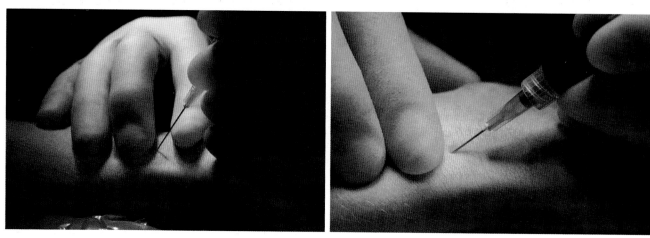

Figure 6.6 Step-by-step guide: sampling the arterial blood gas. (a) Palpating the radial pulse to identify the point of maximal pulsation. (b) Sterilising the area using 2% chlorhexidine in 70% isopropyl alcohol. (c) The skin is punctured at a 45° angle in a proximal direction with the syringe held like a pencil. (d) Flashback followed by syringe filling as the artery is punctured.

Information from a blood gas machine

Firstly, learn where the blood gas machines are in your hospital. Reliable places where they can be found are:

- intensive and high-dependency care areas
- emergency medicine departments
- medical admission wards.

All blood gas analysers should provide the following data set:

- PaO_2
- pH
- $PaCO_2$
- bicarbonate.

Other machines may include electrolytes, haemoglobin, glucose and lactate. Make sure you know which machines do what; there is no point taking an ABG to get a rapid potassium or haemoglobin result and taking it to the wrong machine!

Complications

Pain and discomfort

ABG sampling is painful. The pain is minimised by the practitioner acquiring skill and experience. Patient anxiety is reduced through explanation and reassurance. There is no evidence to suggest topical local anaesthetic is beneficial. Subcutaneous infiltration of a local anaesthetic agent can sting and may distort the anatomy if performed immediately before the procedure.

Haematoma

Natural elasticity of the arterial wall will prevent this, but increasing age and anticoagulant therapy make patients more susceptible. Ensure pressure is applied quickly and check bleeding has stopped before leaving the patient. If necessary ask someone to continue pressure over the puncture site whilst you deal with the sample.

Arteriospasm

Reflex constriction of the artery caused by irritation from the needle can make it difficult to obtain a sample.

Infection and sepsis

This is unlikely if skin is prepared properly. Avoid areas of skin that are inflamed, infected or broken down.

Interpretation of the ABG result

Now you have your sample, you need to be able to interpret the findings. For the normal values of an arterial blood gas see Box 6.3

Box 6.3 **Normal values for blood gas**

- pH 7.35–7.45
- PaO_2 10.5–13.5 kPa (or 80–100 mmHg)
- $PaCO_2$ 4.7–6.0 kPa (or 35–45 mmHg)
- HCO_3^- 22–28 mmol/L
- BE –2 to +2

(although normal ranges may vary slightly between laboratories). There are two initial points to consider. First, is the patient hypoxic? Second, is there an acid–base disturbance? If your blood gas analyser provides other details such as electrolytes, haemoglobin, glucose or lactate then check these too.

Evidence of hypoxaemia

Normal PaO_2 (arterial partial pressure of oxygen) is between 10.5–13.5 kPa: anything below 10.5 and the patient is hypoxic. Hypoxia can be due to ventilation/perfusion mismatch, hypoventilation, abnormal diffusion, or right to left cardiac shunts.

Hypoxia is life-threatening and immediately treatable by increasing the oxygen flow rate or using a higher fixed performance rated device.

Remember to check the inspired oxygen fraction (FiO_2). This is more normally expressed as the percentage of oxygen delivered. Is the PaO_2 disproportionate? For example, with a PaO_2 of 13 kPa on 90% oxygen, the patient is not hypoxic but needing high levels of oxygen to maintain oxygenation – get senior help.

Is there an acid–base disturbance

Many people find acid–base balances confusing but they become easier the more you interpret them. Using Figure 6.7 assess each component. Then ask yourself the following questions.

1 Is there an acidosis or alkalosis?
2 If so, is it respiratory or metabolic in origin?
  - Which component ($PaCO_2$ or HCO_3^-) matches the pH state?
  - $PaCO_2$ reflects a respiratory problem (if high, it may be causing a respiratory acidosis).
  - HCO_3^- reflects a metabolic problem (if low, it suggests a metabolic acidosis).
3 Is there any evidence of compensation?
  - Is the remaining component abnormal in the opposite direction?

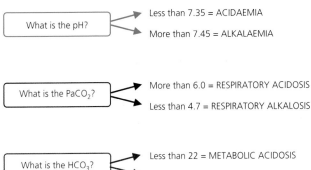

Figure 6.7 Assessing the acid–base disturbance.

Table 6.2 Some common examples of acid–base disturbance.

Respiratory acidosis
Hypoventilation states
Central respiratory depression (e.g. opiates, sedatives, stroke)
Nerve/muscle disorders (e.g. myasthenia gravis, Guillain–Barré)
Lung disorder (e.g. CO_2 retention in COPD, upper airway obstruction)

Respiratory alkalosis
Hyperventilation states
Respiratory (e.g. asthma, pneumonia, pulmonary embolism)
Central causes (e.g. intracerebral haemorrhage, meningitis)
Metabolic (e.g. fever, hyperthyroidism)

Metabolic acidosis
Excess H^+ production – anaerobic respiration in tissues
  (e.g. severe sepsis, intrabdominal pathology)
Inadequate excretion of H^+ – renal failure of any cause, renal tubular
  acidosis, Addisonian crisis
Excess loss of bicarbonate – excessive diarrhoea (e.g. Crohn's disease)
Psychogenic causes (e.g. pain, anxiety)

Metabolic alkalosis
Excess H^+ loss – prolonged vomiting (e.g, pyloric stenosis,
  anorexia nervosa)
Hypokalaemia
Excess reabsorption of bicarbonate – due to excess loss of chloride
  (e.g. prolonged vomiting, use of thiazide and loop diuretics)
Ingestion of acids – not common

- If yes, there is evidence of compensation.
- *Example*: acidosis + high $PaCO_2$ + low HCO_3 = respiratory acidosis with an element of compensation.
- To be fully compensated, the pH needs to be normal.

It may be helpful to evaluate the base excess (BE). This equates to how much base there is left over after balancing out the acid component. If there is a negative base excess this means there is a deficit of base to balance out the acid present – hence the patient has an acidaemia.

Remember, if you are still confused and the numbers are abnormal do not hesitate to ask for help. For some common causes of acid–base disturbance see Table 6.2.

An ABG example

A 17-year-old boy with known asthma presents to the emergency department with an acute exacerbation. This ABG was taken on room air:

pH   7.50
PaO_2 10.0 kPa
$PaCO_2$ 1.3 kPa
HCO_3^- 24 mmol/L

1 Is the patient hypoxic?
  Yes. A PaO_2 of 10 kPa is abnormally low, particularly for a young man. Oxygen should be administered, initially at high flow and preferably humidified.
2 Is acidosis or alkalosis present?
  This ABG shows an alkalaemia, with a higher than normal pH.
3 What is the cause of the acid–base disturbance?
  This is matched by a low $PaCO_2$, so he has a respiratory alkalosis.

If this sample was taken on 40% oxygen the PaO_2 result should be interpreted differently. It would be disproportionate to the inspired oxygen concentration, and with the clinical picture there should be a low threshold for ITU review.

Further ABGs should be obtained. Life-threatening asthma is said to be present when the PaO_2 is below 8 kPa and the $PaCO_2$ moves into the normal range or higher. In this situation, the patient is hypoxic and is beginning to tire and may be in need of respiratory support.

Asthma is a disease which still has a high mortality rate, especially in young people, so have a low threshold for senior review.

Handy hints/troubleshooting

- Compensation for metabolic acidosis is through hyperventilation, in diabetic ketoacidosis (DKA) patients who have a rising CO_2 are tiring and are dangerously unwell.
- Remember the inspired oxygen (FiO_2) when interpreting the PaO_2.
- Patients will die from hypoxia before hypercarbia; don't be scared of giving oxygen.
- In a patient with a good radial pulse, call for help if you have missed it twice.
- In a patient with a weak pulse, think about the calling the emergency medical/arrest team.
- Find a patient label before taking the sample and jot down the patient's inspired oxygen and temperature.

Further reading

Driscoll P, Brown TA, Gwinnutt CL, Wardle T. (1997) *A Simple Guide to Blood Gas Analysis*. BMJ Publishing Group, London.

Hennessy I, Japp A. (2007) *Arterial Blood Gases Made Easy*. Churchill Livingstone, Edinburgh.

Longmore M, Wilkinson I, Torok E. (2001) *Oxford Handbook of Clinical Medicine*, 5th edn. Oxford University Press, Oxford.

CHAPTER 7

Sampling: Lumbar Puncture

Mike Byrne

Birmingham Heartlands Hospital, Birmingham, UK

OVERVIEW

By the end of this chapter you should have a good understanding of:
- indications and contraindications of lumbar puncture (LP)
- anatomical considerations
- different types of spinal needles
- the practical procedure of LP
- possible complications and their management
- interpretation of results for meningitis.

Introduction

Lumbar puncture (LP) is an infrequently performed procedure that has an important role in the diagnosis and treatment of many serious conditions. A full understanding of the anatomy and contraindications is essential if potentially life-threatening complications are to be avoided.

Indications

You are most likely to encounter lumbar puncture on the acute medical wards for the diagnosis of meningitis or subarachnoid haemorrhage. Its indications are:

Diagnostic
- CNS infection (e.g. bacterial, viral, TB meningitis)
- subarachnoid haemorrhage
- neurological disease (e.g. multiple sclerosis, Guillain–Barré syndrome).

Therapeutic
- intrathecal chemotherapy
- removal of CSF (e.g. idiopathic intracranial hypertension).

Anaesthetic
- spinal anaesthesia for lower limb/lower abdominal surgery.

Box 7.1 **Lumbar puncture and anticoagulation**

Patient on full anticoagulation:
- warfarin – stop and ensure INR <1.5
- unfractionated heparin infusion – stop infusion and ensure APTT normal (after approx 4 h)

Prophylactic anticoagulation:
- unfractionated heparin – wait 4 h after dose, can give heparin 1 h after LP
- low molecular weight heparin – wait 12 hours after dose, can give 4 hours after LP

Platelets – ensure >80 × 10³

Aspirin/NSAIDs – no increased risk of spinal/epidural haematoma

Contraindications

These can be absolute or relative.

Absolute
- Patient refusal.
- Clotting abnormality or full therapeutic anticoagulation. Risk of epidural haematoma causing cord compression (see Box 7.1 for timing of LP if anticoagulation has been given).
- Raised intracranial pressure (ICP) (risk of 'coning'). If raised ICP is suspected (see Box 7.2 for symptoms and signs) then a CT scan should be performed before LP to look for hydrocephalus or a space-occupying lesion. Unfortunately a CT scan is not infallible so the indication for LP should be strong.
- Local infection at injection site. Risks causing epidural abscess or meningitis.

Relative
- Systemic sepsis. Risks causing epidural abscess or meningitis.
- Neurological disease. Any subsequent new neurological symptoms can be blamed on the LP. The indication needs to be strong, the patient's informed consent given and a full neurological examination should be performed and documented before LP.

Anatomy

Lumbar puncture requires the insertion of a needle into the cerebrospinal fluid (CSF) in the lumbar region of the spine (Figure 7.1). In adults the spinal cord ends at the lower border of

ABC of Practical Procedures. Edited by T. Nutbeam and R. Daniels. © 2010 Blackwell Publishing, ISBN: 978-1-4051-8595-0.

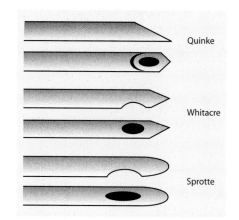

Figure 7.2 Spinal needles.

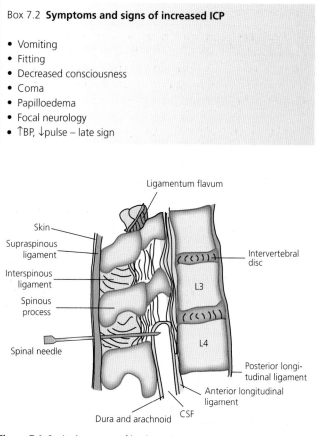

Figure 7.1 Sagittal anatomy of lumbar spine.

L1 (L3 in children), and so insertion of the needle must be below this level to avoid possible spinal cord injury.

The spinal cord is surrounded by the three meninges which stretch from the foramen magnum to the sacral level (S2). The dura mater forms a tough fibroelastic outer layer with the arachnoid mater attached to it beneath. There is then a space, the subarachnoid space, before the pia mater which is closely adherent to the cord itself. The CSF is located within this subarachnoid space. The pia mater extends caudally as the filum terminale and anchors the spinal cord and dura to the coccyx.

In order to reach the subarachnoid space the lumbar puncture needle needs to pass through skin, subcutaneous tissue, vertebral ligaments, the dura and the arachnoid mater. The ligaments are the supraspinous ligament running between the tips of the vertebral spines, the interspinous ligament stretching between adjacent spines, and the ligamentum flavum which forms a tough ligament that connects adjacent laminae. The dura lies immediately deep to the ligamentum flavum, although there is a potential space between these structures that can be expanded by injecting fluid or air. This is the epidural space and is where the catheter for an epidural anaesthetic is inserted.

Equipment

Lumbar puncture requires specialised spinal needles (Figure 7.2) which are long and relatively narrow gauge (18–29G). They differ

in the shape of the tip of the needle and in the location of the opening at the tip. The different designs have been produced to try to reduce the incidence of postdural puncture headache (see 'Complications'). The pencil point tips of the Whitacre and Sprotte needles are designed to split apart the fibres of the dura on insertion, rather than cutting a hole in them. This allows the fibres to come together again on needle withdrawal, sealing the hole and preventing further CSF leakage which can lead to headache.

The narrower-gauge spinal needles have an introducer to pass the needle through. This helps to prevent the needle bending too much on insertion and not following the desired course.

Stylets are included to add stiffness to the needle for insertion and block the opening at the needle tip so that it doesn't become blocked with skin or subcutaneous tissue during insertion.

Patient positioning

Lumbar puncture can be performed with the patient sitting or lying in a lateral position. The sitting position allows easier identification of the midline (especially in obese patients where the vertebral spines can be difficult or impossible to feel); however, the patient may be too ill to sit up.

Both positions require the patient to flex their lumbar spine so that the intervertebral spaces open up maximally to allow easier needle passage. This is achieved by asking the patient to put their chin on their chest, bring their knees as far up to their chest as they can and push their lumbar spine backwards.

For the sitting position, ask the patient to sit on the bed with their feet placed on a stool, adjusting the height of the bed or stool until the patient's hips are adequately flexed. Ask them to lean forward over a pillow to produce arching of the back (Figure 7.3).

For the lateral position, ask the patient to lie on their left side if you are right-handed and vice versa, with their head supported on a pillow so that their spine is in a horizontal line. Their back should be along the edge of the bed and must be perpendicular to the bed in the vertical plane. Then ask them to curl up as described above (Figure 7.4).

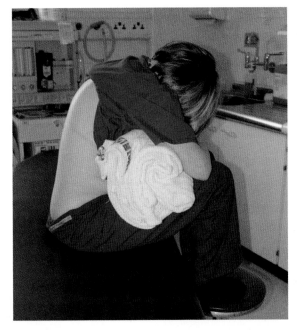

Figure 7.3 Sitting position.

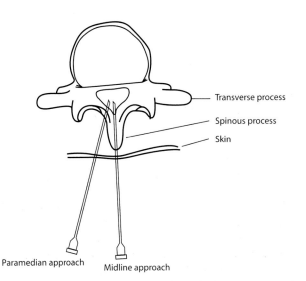

Figure 7.4 Lateral position.

Procedure

The midline or the paramedian approach can be used (Figure 7.5). The midline approach is easier to learn and is successful in the majority of cases. The paramedian approach can be useful in difficult cases where bony osteophytes, calcified ligaments or narrowed intervertebral spaces obstruct a midline approach.

Step-by-step guide: lumbar puncture
Midline approach
1 Obtain informed consent.
2 Prepare equipment (see Box 7.3 and Figure 7.6).
3 Position the patient (see 'Patient positioning' above).
4 Scrub up – wear mask, hat, sterile gown and gloves. You will see the procedure performed with sterile gloves only but this is bad practice. An epidural abscess can leave a patient paralysed!
5 Sterilise the skin of the patient's lower back with a spirit-based antiseptic (2% chlorhexidine or betadine) (Figure 7.7a) and prepare a sterile field with drapes covering the anterior superior iliac spines so that Tuffier's line (L3–L4 level) can be identified without desterilising oneself (Figure 7.7b).

Box 7.3 **Equipment for lumbar puncture**

- Sterile gown and gloves, mask and hat
- Sterile pack – with gauze, galley pot
- Sterile drapes
- Chlorhexidine/betadine in spirit
- Lidocaine 1%
- 5-mL syringe
- 25G needle (orange)
- Spinal needle
- Manometer
- Three-way tap
- Collection tubes: three sterile universal containers + glucose tube (fluoride/grey top)

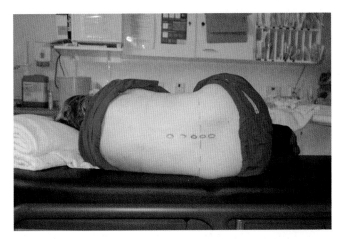

Figure 7.5 Midline and paramedian approaches to lumbar puncture.

Transverse process
Spinous process
Skin

Paramedian approach
Midline approach

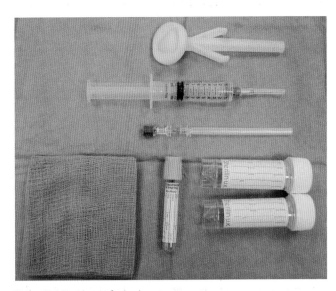

Figure 7.6 Equipment for lumbar puncture.

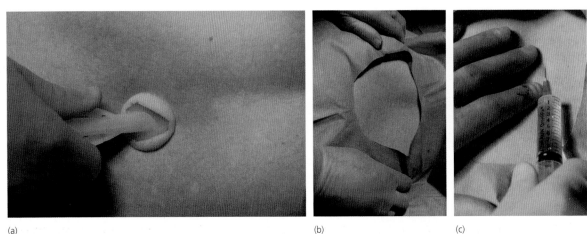

(a)　　　　　　　　　　　　　　　　　(b)　　　　　　　　　(c)

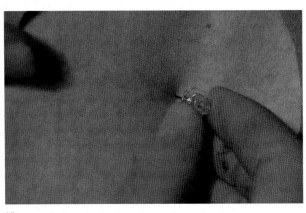

(d)

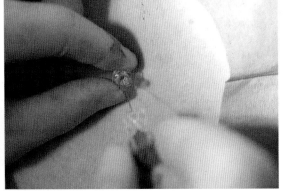

(e)

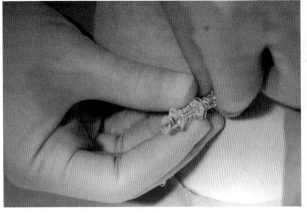

(f)　　　　　　　　　　　　　　　　　(g)

Figure 7.7 Step-by-step guide: lumbar puncture. (a) Sterilising the area with 2% chlorhexidine solution. (b) Palpating the iliac crests to identify landmarks. (c) Using a blue needle to infiltrate local anaesthetic. (d) Inserting an introducer needle. (e) Inserting the spinal needle through the introducer. (f) CSF flashback through spinal needle. (g) Assistant collecting CSF.

6 Identify the L3/L4 interspace (Figure 7.8) and raise a subcutaneous wheal with 1% lidocaine using an orange (25G) or blue (23G) needle. Inject a further 1–2 mL into the subcutaneous space (Figure 7.7c). Allow time for the lidocaine to work.

7 With your non-dominant hand grip the spinous process of L3 between thumb and index or middle finger. This anchors the skin and allows easier identification of the midline.

8 Insert the needle (or introducer if narrow-gauge needle used) at 90° to the skin in the midline at the middle to the cephalad end of the interspace (Figure 7.7d,e). If a non-pencil point needle is used insert with the bevel facing laterally (in the same direction as the fibres of the dura) so as to encourage parting of the dural fibres rather than cutting them. This decreases the risk of post-dural puncture headache.

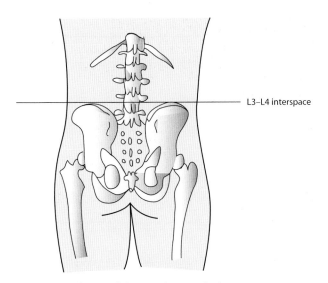
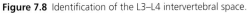

L3–L4 interspace

Figure 7.8 Identification of the L3–L4 intervertebral space.

9 Advance the needle slowly. You will get feedback of the needle's progress as it passes through the ligaments, and often feel a pop or click as the resistance from the ligamentum flavum and dura is overcome at a depth of approximately 4–6 cm (may be shallower or deeper in particularly slim or obese patients). Stop advancing the needle and withdraw the stylet. The CSF should flow freely (Figure 7.7f). Note that even with definite dural puncture it can take a few seconds for the CSF flow to be seen, especially if narrower gauge needles are used and the patient is in the lateral position.

10 If bony resistance is felt on advancing the needle, withdraw the needle and introducer back to the subcutaneous tissue, redirect them about 15° cephalad and reinsert. Continue to repeat this manoeuvre if further bony contact is met. If this manoeuvre is not successful check the patient's position and ensure your needle insertion and advancement are in the midline. It can be easy to stray from the midline especially with the patient in the lateral position. If this fails, repeat the whole procedure at the L4/L5 interspace. Do not attempt lumbar puncture at L2/L3 or above as spinal cord damage has been reported.

11 If you still encounter problems the paramedian approach can be attempted, or seek help from a more senior member of the team. For those patients that still present a challenge, seek assistance from clinicians who regularly perform lumbar punctures – the neurologists and anaesthetists.

Paramedian approach

1 After local anaesthesia, insert the needle 1–2 cm lateral to the upper border of the spinous process perpendicular to the skin. Bony resistance will be felt as the vertebral lamina is contacted.

2 Withdraw the needle slightly and reinsert, aiming approximately 15° medially and 30° cephalad. The needle should now pass over the vertebral lamina and a pop will be felt as the dura is punctured.

Sampling

1 Once lumbar puncture is successful it is possible to measure the CSF pressure by attaching a manometer via a three-way tap to

---

Box 7.4 **Postdural puncture headache**

Following LP continued leak of CSF through the dural puncture site can lead to traction on the cranial meninges. This can cause a headache with the following characteristics:
- constant
- dull
- occipital or bifrontal
- postural – relieved by lying down; worse on sitting or standing
- meningism may be present
- onset is usually within 24–48 hours of LP
- 30% incidence with 22G needle
- 1% incidence with 26G needle.

Risk is minimised by using atraumatic needles (Whitacre, Sprotte) of small gauge, but CSF collection can take a long time if needles smaller than 22G are used. There is no evidence that the amount of CSF taken or lying flat after LP reduces the risk.

Management involves rest, oral analgesics and maintaining hydration. All cases will resolve with time but if symptoms are severe, liaise with an anaesthetist to consider an epidural blood patch. For this 20 mL of the patient's blood is taken from a vein under aseptic conditions and injected into the epidural space at the level of the LP. This blood will clot and plug the hole preventing further CSF leak. Immediate relief is obtained in >90% of cases.

the end of the needle. Normal value is 5–20 cmH$_2$O with the patient in the lateral position.

2 Collect 5–10 drops (approx 1 mL) of CSF into three sequentially numbered universal containers and also into a fluoride tube (grey top) for glucose measurement (Figure 7.7g).

3 Remove the needle and apply a dressing.

4 Send samples for appropriate investigations. For suspected meningitis send for urgent microscopy, culture, protein and glucose (send blood for plasma glucose measurement as well).

5 Other possible tests include cytology, virology, TB culture, syphilis serology, oligoclonal bands and xanthochromia.

6 Monitor the patient's CNS observations and blood pressure regularly. Be aware of the possibility of a postdural puncture headache (Box 7.4).

Complications

Back pain—Localised soft tissue trauma at injection site is common and may last a few days.

Postdural puncture headache (PDPH)—See Box 7.4.

Neurological sequelae—Temporary symptoms of paraesthesia or motor weakness may result from needle damage or stretching of a nerve root. The majority resolve within a few weeks. Permanent neurological damage is extremely rare (less than 1 in 10 000) and should be assessed by a neurologist.

Infection—Meningitis, encephalitis or epidural abscess are very rare but can result if strict aseptic technique is not followed. If focal neurology develops and an epidural abscess is suspected then an urgent MRI is necessary to confirm the diagnosis followed by emergency neurosurgical drainage. Antimicrobials are given as appropriate.

Table 7.1 Typical CSF in meningitis.

	Normal	Bacterial	Viral	Tuberculosis
Pressure	5–20 cm CSF	Often ↑	Often ↑	Often ↑
Appearance	Clear	Turbid/purulent	Clear	Turbid
Predominant cell	Nil	Neutrophils	Lymphocytes	Lymphocytes
Lymphocytes	<5/mm^3	<50/mm^3	50–500/mm^3	100–1000/mm^3
Neutrophils	0	>200/mm^3	0	<200/mm^3
Protein	0.1–0.4 g/L	>1.5 g/L	<1 g/L	1–5 g/L
Glucose	2–4 mmol/L >50% plasma glucose	<50% plasma glucose	>50% plasma glucose	<50% plasma glucose
Gram stain	Normal	May show organisms	Normal	Normal

Haematoma—A spinal subdural or epidural haematoma can cause spinal cord compression and requires urgent MRI and emergency neurosurgical drainage.

Cerebellar tonsillar herniation (coning)—In the presence of increased ICP the cerebellar tonsils may be forced through the foramen magnum, resulting in compression of the medulla and neurological deterioration or death.

Interpretation of results

See Table 7.1.

Blood in CSF – subarachnoid haemorrhage or bloody tap?

Bloody tap is suggested by:
- drop in RBC count in successive collection tubes
- no xanthochromia – yellow supernatant on spun CSF.

Causes of increased CSF protein

↑Protein	↑↑Protein
Bacterial meningitis	Severe bacterial meningitis
Multiple sclerosis	Tuberculosis
Guillain–Barré syndrome	Spinal tumours
Acoustic neuroma	

Handy hints/troubleshooting

- Patient positioning is key – take the time to get this right.
- Spend time obtaining consent and discussing the procedure with the patient – this should alleviate their fears and allow them to help you by optimal positioning.
- Be absolutely sure that you are in the midline, especially with overweight patients.
- Ensure your assistant is well prepared, with bottles open, labelled and in the correct order.
- If you want to exclude infection, remember to take a venous blood glucose level for comparison to the CSF result.

Further reading

Boon JM, Abrahams PH, Meiring JH, Welch T. (2004) Lumbar punctures: anatomical review of a clinical skill. *Clin Anat* 17: 544–53.

Ellenby MS, Tegtmeyer K, Lai S, Braner DAV. (2006) Lumbar puncture. *N Engl J Med* 355: e12.

Evans RW. (1998) Complications of lumbar puncture. *Neurol Clin* 16: 83–105.

Hasbun R, Abrahams J, Jekel J, Quagliarello VJ. (2001) Computed tomography of the head before lumbar puncture in adults with suspected meningitis. *N Engl J Med* 345: 1727.

Kneen R, Solomon T, Appleton R. (2002) The role of lumbar puncture in suspected CNS infection – a disappearing skill? *Arch Dis Child* 87: 181–3.

Straus S, Thorpe K. (2006) How do I perform a lumbar puncture and analyze the results to diagnose bacterial meningitis? *JAMA* 296: 2012–22.

Van de Beek D, de Gans J, Tunkel AR, Wijdicks EFM. (2006) Community-acquired bacterial meningitis in adults. *N Engl J Med* 354: 44.

CHAPTER 8

Sampling: Ascitic Tap

Andrew King

Centre for Liver Research, University of Birmingham, Birmingham, UK

OVERVIEW

By the end of this chapter you should be able to:
- understand the indications for performing an ascitic tap
- be able to examine for and assess the extent of ascites
- describe how to perform an ascitic tap
- interpret the results of an ascitic tap.

Introduction

Indications

Evaluation of new-onset ascites

A diagnostic ascitic tap is a crucial part of the work-up of a patient with new-onset ascites. Analysis of the fluid can help decide the most appropriate further investigations to perform in order to determine the cause of the ascites.

Assessment of established ascites

In patients with established ascites who have an unexplained change in clinical condition, an ascitic tap is essential to investigate for the presence of spontaneous bacterial peritonitis. Assessment of protein concentration can also indicate new pathology (e.g. raised protein concentration in Budd–Chiari syndrome on a background of chronic liver disease).

Contraindications

A diagnostic ascitic tap should not be attempted in the presence of the following conditions:
- acute abdomen requiring surgical intervention
- urinary retention/distended bladder
- pregnancy
- abdominal wall infection
- extensive adhesions
- dilated loops of bowel (e.g. volvulus).

If required, it may be possible to perform a tap under direct vision using ultrasound guidance.

ABC of Practical Procedures. Edited by T. Nutbeam and R. Daniels. © 2010
Blackwell Publishing, ISBN: 978-1-4051-8595-0.

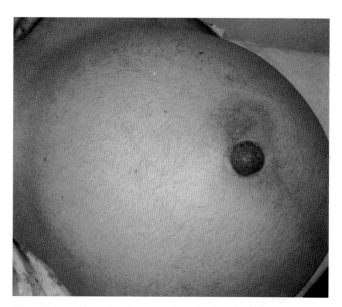

Figure 8.1 A patient with an obvious distended abdomen.

Coagulopathy

- Many patients who require a diagnostic ascitic tap have chronic liver disease with deranged clotting. There is evidence that performing a **diagnostic** tap with a small gauge needle (e.g. a green needle) is safe in the presence of low platelets or elevated INR/PT.
- In the presence of active fibrinolysis or DIC a diagnostic tap should not be attempted.

Clinical detection of ascites

Ascites is the accumulation of fluid within the peritoneal cavity. The presence of ascites can usually only be confirmed clinically at volumes greater than 1500 mL. It is significantly more difficult to reliably detect ascites in those with central obesity.

Initial inspection is important, as the shape of the abdomen will give clues as to the presence of ascites. With the patient supine, accumulated fluid will cause bulging of the flanks; on standing the fluid will accumulate in the lower abdomen and pelvis (Figure 8.1). Bulging of the flanks may also be caused by subcutaneous fat in obese patients; further examination is required to distinguish fat from fluid.

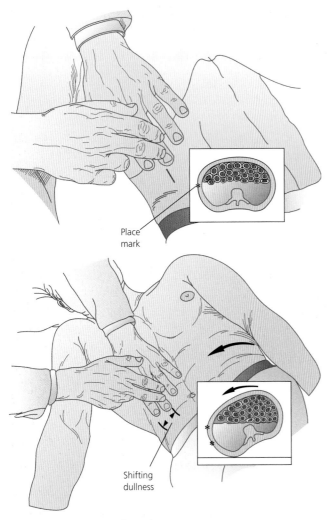

Place
mark

Shifting
dullness

Figure 8.2 How to percuss for ascites.

The most reliable clinical sign is the presence of shifting dull-ness. Fluid within the abdomen will accumulate in the lowest, most dependent region. Conversely, gas-filled, less dense loops of bowel will float on top of the fluid and accumulate in the highest region.

Detecting shifting dullness (Figure 8.2)

1 Position patient in the supine position.
2 Percuss from the umbilicus and move laterally down the abdom-inal wall towards yourself.
3 Stop at the point of transition from tympanic to dull percussion.
4 Keep your fingers or mark this position and ask the patient to roll towards you.
5 Pause briefly to allow the fluid to shift within the abdomen.
6 Positive test: when ascites is present, the area of dullness will shift to the dependent side. The area of tympany will shift towards the top.

Anatomy

When performing a diagnostic ascitic tap the patient should be in the supine position with the head of the bed slightly elevated to allow fluid to accumulate in the lower abdomen.

Box 8.1 Equipment for ascitic tap

- Sterile gloves and gown
- Dressing pack containing gauze and sterile drape
- Antiseptic skin preparation
- 5 mL 1% lidocaine
- 25 G (orange) needle
- 21 G (green) needle × 2
- 10-mL syringe
- 20-mL syringe
- Adhesive dressing
- Universal containers × 3
- Blood culture bottles × 1 set

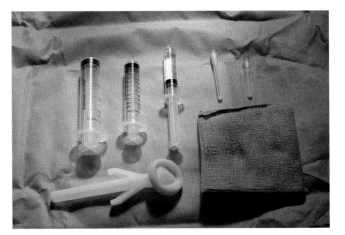

Figure 8.3 The equipment required for ascitic tap.

The ideal site for a diagnostic tap is in the area of flank dullness in the lower left or right quadrant of the abdomen. Depending on patient size this is typically 5 cm superior and medial to the anterior superior iliac spine.

It is important to remember that the inferior epigastric vessels run adjacent to the rectus abdominis muscles and therefore the site should be as far lateral as possible to avoid vascular damage.

Avoid superficial veins and surgical scars, as they may have collateral vessels or underlying adherent bowel.

Step-by-step guide: ascitic tap

Give a full explanation to the patient in simple terms and ensure they consent to the procedure.
- Set up your trolley (Box 8.1 and Figure 8.3).
- **Prepare your trolley as a sterile field. Wear a plastic disposable apron and non-sterile gloves, and take alcohol hand rub with you.**

1 Ensure the patient is comfortable, lying with the head of the bed slightly elevated and with an empty bladder.
2 Percuss the ascites and mark the selected site (as above).
3 Wash hands thoroughly, put on sterile gloves and a gown and clean the area with antiseptic fluid (e.g. 2% chlorhexidine in 70% isopropyl alcohol) (Figure 8.4a).

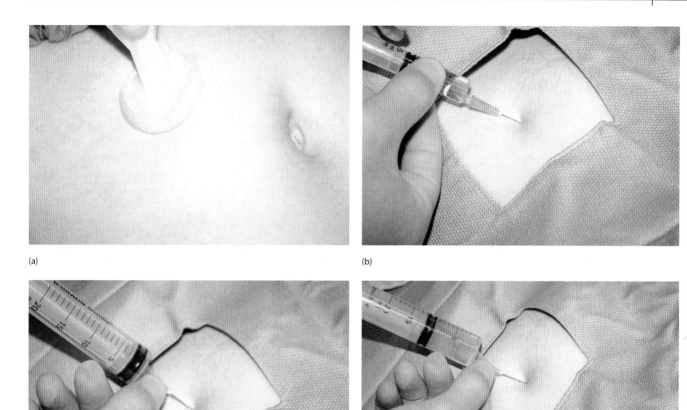

(a)

(b)

(c)

(d)

Figure 8.4 Step-by-step guide: ascitic tap. (a) Cleaning the area (2% chlorhexidine in 70% alcohol). (b) Infiltration of local anaesthetic. (c) Aspirating whilst advancing the green needle. (d) Successful aspiration of peritoneal fluid (the needle is not advanced any further).

4 Infiltrate the skin at the chosen site with local anaesthetic (e.g. 1% lidocaine), using an orange needle and 10-mL syringe (Figure 8.4b).

5 Use a green needle to infiltrate the deeper subcutaneous tissues; a 'flashback' of ascitic fluid will occur when the peritoneal space is reached.

6 Using a green needle and 20-mL syringe, insert the needle perpendicular to the skin and slowly advance. Aspirate gently as you advance the needle until fluid can be easily aspirated (Figure 8.4c).

7 Aspirate 20 mL fluid and withdraw the needle (Figure 8.4d).

8 Apply pressure to the site and cover with an adhesive dressing.

9 Distribute the aspirate into the containers described in Table 8.1, ensuring sterility throughout.

Analysis of ascitic fluid

Biochemistry

Fluid protein and fluid albumin concentrations will identify the fluid as either a transudate or exudate. Exudates are usually caused by inflammatory conditions such as malignancy and

Table 8.1 Samples required from diagnostic tap.

	Specimen	Tests requested
Biochemistry	Universal container	Fluid protein Fluid albumin
Microbiology	Sterile universal container (for Gram stain and cell count) Blood culture bottles (for culture and sensitivities) EDTA blood tube (for cell count if sample heavily bloodstained)	M, C and S Cell count
Cytology	Universal container	Cytology

M, C and S, microscopy, cultures and sensitivities.

infection. Transudates result from reduced plasma oncotic pressure or increased plasma hydrostatic pressure:

- total protein concentration: transudate <30 g/L; exudate >30 g/L.

Total protein concentration alone is an unreliable method as, for example, cardiac ascites may have a high protein content,

Table 8.2 Causes of ascites classified as transudate and exudate.

Transudate (protein <30 g/L; SAAG >11 g/L)	Exudate (protein >30g/L; SAAG <11 g/L)
Cirrhosis	Malignancy
Chronic liver disease	Pancreatitis
Congestive cardiac failure	Peritoneal tuberculosis
Constrictive pericarditis	Nephrotic syndrome
	Chylous ascites

and normal peritoneal fluid has a protein concentration of 40 g/L.

Calculation of the serum ascites albumin gradient (SAAG) is a more reliable method of determining whether the fluid is a transudate or exudate:

- SAAG = [serum albumin] − [ascitic fluid albumin]; transudate >11 g/L; exudate <11 g/L.

Table 8.2 describes causes of exudative and transudative ascites.

Microbiology

A cell count can be performed rapidly and is the single best test for the detection of spontaneous bacterial peritonitis (SBP):

- neutrophil count > 250 cells/microlitre = SBP.

SBP is often associated with low concentrations of bacteria. The rate of detection can be increased by the direct inoculation of blood culture bottles with ascitic fluid at the bedside.

Cytology

The presence of malignant cells in ascitic fluid confirms the diagnosis of malignancy, but it is important to remember that the absence of malignant cells does not exclude malignancy. Liver metastases and primary hepatocellular carcinoma are unlikely to provide positive findings.

Potential complications

Failure to obtain sample—If it is not possible to obtain a sample, repeating at a different site or changing sides may help. If it is still not possible, then an ultrasound scan should be performed and either a site marked for aspiration or a sample obtained under direct ultrasound guidance.

Persistent leakage from site of tap—If necessary apply a stoma bag to the site until leakage stops.

Abdominal wall haematoma—The risk is higher with deranged clotting, but most resolve spontaneously.

Significant haemorrhage and perforation—These are extremely rare complications of diagnostic ascitic tap if it performed correctly. They may result if bowel is adherent to the abdominal wall or if there is significant collateral vessel within abdominal wall. Seek senior help.

Handy hints/troubleshooting

- Take time to position your patient correctly and identify your landmarks.
- Occasionally, you may only be able to aspirate a few mL of fluid – in this case, ask the lab how much fluid is needed for each test and prioritise tests according to clinical suspicion.
- Consider using an ultrasound-guided technique if the blind technique is unsuccessful or if there are particular concerns.

Further reading

Hoefs JC. (1990) Diagnostic paracentesis: a potent clinical tool. *Gastroenterology* 98: 230–6.

Jeffery J, Murphy M. (2008) Ascitic fluid analysis. *Hosp Med* 62(5): 282–6.

Mallory A, Schaefer J. (1978) Complications of diagnostic paracentesis in patients with liver disease. *JAMA* 239(7): 628–30.

Moore K, Aithal G. (2006) British Society of Gastroenterology Guidelines on the management of ascites in cirrhosis. *Gut* 55: 1–12.

Runyon B, Canawati H, Akriviadis E. (1988) Optimisation of ascitic fluid culture technique. *Gastroenterology* 95: 1351–5.

Runyon B, Montano A, Akriviadis E *et al.* (1992) The serum ascites albumin gradient is superior to the exudates–transudate concept in the diagnosis of ascites. *Ann Intern Med* 117: 215–20.

Williams J, Simel D. (1992) Does this patient have ascites? *JAMA* 267(19): 2645–8.

Wong C, Holroyd-Leduc J, Thorpe K *et al.* (2008) Does this patient have bacterial peritonitis or portal hypertension? *JAMA* 299(10): 1166–78.

CHAPTER 9

Sampling: Pleural Aspiration

Nicola Sinden

West Midlands Rotation, Birmingham, UK

OVERVIEW

By the end of this chapter you should be able to:
- understand the indications and contraindications for pleural aspiration
- identify and understand the relevant anatomy
- describe the procedure of performing a pleural aspiration
- clinically assess a pleural effusion
- understand the difference between and the causes of transudative and exudative pleural effusions.

Indications

Pleural aspiration may be:
- diagnostic (to determine the cause of a pleural effusion)
- therapeutic (to relieve symptoms of dyspnoea).

Contraindications (relative)

- Small volumes of fluid or fluid difficult to detect by examination (an ultrasound scan of the thorax with marking of a site for aspiration can be helpful in these situations).
- Deranged INR (ideally INR should be less than 1.5).
- Severe underlying lung disease (complications of the procedure may be life-threatening).

Anatomy

The pleurae

The pleurae are really one continuous membrane which lines the inner surface of the thoracic cavity and diaphragm (parietal pleura) and covers the lungs (visceral pleura). Between this double layer lies the pleural cavity. In pathological states this potential space can expand and fill with excess liquid (pleural effusion; Figure 9.1) or air (pneumothorax).

The intercostal muscles and the neurovascular bundle

The intercostal space between adjacent ribs is filled by the intercostal muscles. The intercostal muscles are composed of several

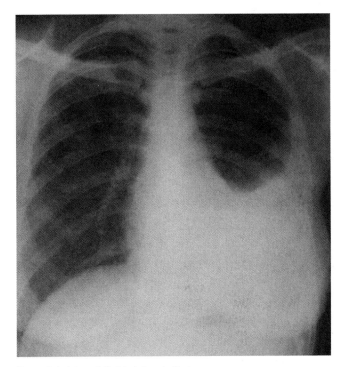

Figure 9.1 A large left-sided pleural effusion.

layers with the muscle fibres running in different directions. Lying between the innermost and the inner intercostal muscles is the neurovascular bundle. The neurovascular bundle contains the vein, artery and nerve (Figure 9.2a). It is imperative to avoid this bundle when performing a pleural aspiration. The chances of penetrating this bundle can be minimised by always inserting the needle over the upper border of a rib rather than under (Figure 9.2b).

Step-by-step guide: pleural aspiration

- **Give a full explanation to the patient in simple terms and ensure they consent to the procedure.**
- **Set up your trolley (Box 9.1). Figure 9.3 shows the equipment required for a diagnostic aspiration.**
- **Prepare your trolley as a sterile field. Wear a plastic disposable apron and sterile gloves, and take alcohol hand rub with you.**

ABC of Practical Procedures. Edited by T. Nutbeam and R. Daniels. © 2010 Blackwell Publishing, ISBN: 978-1-4051-8595-0.

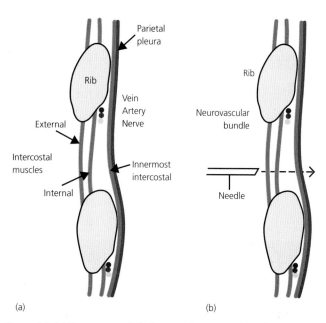

Parietal
pleura

Rib

External

Intercostal
muscles

Internal

Vein
Artery
Nerve

Innermost
intercostal

Rib

Neurovascular
bundle

Needle

(a)

(b)

Figure 9.2 (a) The anatomy of the intercostal nerves and vessels.
(b) Insertion of needle over rib to avoid damage to neurovascular bundle.

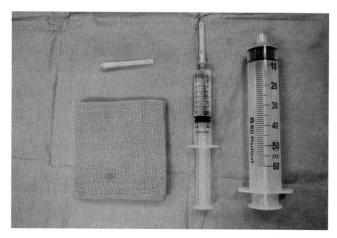

Figure 9.3 Equipment for performing a diagnostic pleural aspiration.

Box 9.1 **Equipment for diagnostic pleural aspiration**

- Dressing pack and solution (we recommend 2% chlorhexidine in 70% isopropyl alcohol) for cleansing of the skin
- Sterile gloves and gown
- 1 or 2% lidocaine
- 10-mL syringe for local anaesthetic
- One blue needle
- Two green needles
- 50-mL syringe
- Specimen containers as clinically indicated, usually three white top universal containers, one glucose (fluoride oxalate) bottle, ABG syringe, blood culture bottles
- Skin dressing for post procedure

1 Firstly confirm the site and size of the pleural effusion by clinical examination and review of the chest X-ray (CXR).

2 Ideally ask the patient to sit on the edge of their bed and lean forwards placing their elbows onto a pillow placed on the bedside table. Alternatively sit the patient up in bed.

3 Percuss the chest posteriorly to determine the level of the effusion. Mark a site on the posterior chest wall medial to the angle of the scapula and one intercostal space below the upper limit of dullness to percussion.

4 Use a strict aseptic technique. Wear sterile gloves and gown and consider face mask with visor.

5 Prepare the skin with antiseptic solution and allow to dry, and apply a sterile drape (Figure 9.4a).

6 Infiltrate the skin with local anaesthetic using a blue (23G) needle or orange (25G) needle (Figure 9.4b). Then use a green needle (21G) to infiltrate deeper. The needle should be inserted just above the upper border of the rib to avoid the intercostal neurovascular bundle. Always aspirate before injecting local anaesthetic to ensure that you are not in a blood vessel. Usually

you should be able to aspirate pleural fluid with the full length of a green (21G) needle.

Diagnostic pleural aspiration (tap)

For a diagnostic pleural tap attach a green needle to the 50-mL syringe and insert the needle through the area of skin which has been anaesthetised (Figure 9.4c). Again, the needle should be inserted just above the upper border of the rib. Aspirate 50 mL of pleural fluid then withdraw the needle and apply a dressing to the site.

Therapeutic pleural aspiration (Figures 9.5 and 9.6)

Some hospitals have ready-made pleural aspiration packs.

Otherwise, in addition to the equipment listed in Box 9.1 you will need:
- large-bore IV cannula – 14G (brown/orange) or 16G (grey)
- three-way tap
- IV giving set
- sterile container/bag for collection of fluid.

7 Initially verify that the insertion site is correct by aspirating fluid with a green needle. If unable to aspirate fluid with a green needle then get an ultrasound of the chest to confirm the location of fluid and ask the radiologist to leave a mark on the skin.

8 When the position has been confirmed, insert the large-bore cannula into the area of skin that has been anaesthetised until a flashback of pleural fluid is seen. Then withdraw the needle whilst advancing the cannula into the pleural space. As the needle is withdrawn, place your sterile-gloved thumb over the end of the cannula to prevent air entering the pleural cavity.

9 Attach the three-way tap to the end of the cannula and attach the 50-mL syringe to the opposite port (Figure 9.4d).

10 Attach the IV giving set to the side port of the three-way tap and place the other end of the giving set into the sterile container or bag for collection of the pleural fluid.

11 Aspirate the pleural fluid 50 mL at a time, moving the three-way tap to empty the syringe into the container or bag. Do not remove more than 1.5 L of fluid due to the risk of re-expansion pulmonary oedema.

12 At the end of the procedure ask the patient to breathe out, remove the cannula and apply a dressing to the site.

13 Request a chest X-ray post procedure.

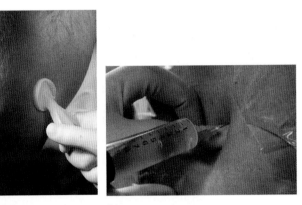
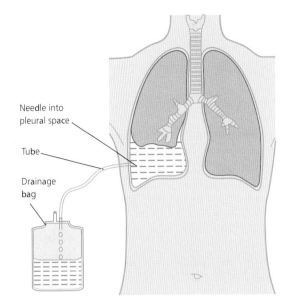

(a)

(b)

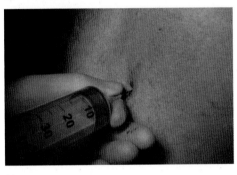

(c)

Needle into
pleural space

Tube

Drainage
bag

Figure 9.6 Therapeutic pleural aspiration.

Pleural fluid analysis

Note the pleural fluid appearance (e.g. serous, blood tinged, frank blood or purulent). Send the pleural fluid for the following investigations.

Microbiology

- Approximately 15 mL of fluid.
- Send fluid in a white top universal container for microscopy, cultures and sensitivities (M, C & S), and for acid/alcohol-fast bacilli (AAFB) and *Mycobacterium tuberculosis* (TB) culture.
- Sending some additional fluid in blood culture bottles increases the yield, especially for anaerobic organisms.

Biochemistry

- Approximately 15 mL of fluid.
- Send fluid in a white top universal container for protein and lactate dehydrogenase (LDH).
- Send fluid in a grey top (fluoride oxalate) bottle for glucose (low in infection and rheumatoid arthritis).
- With an empyema the pleural fluid may appear purulent – do not put these samples into a blood gas analyser. Non-purulent fluid can be put into an ABG syringe and the pH checked. A pleural fluid pH of <7.2 suggests an empyema or parapneumonic effusion.

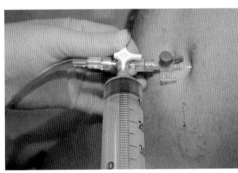

(d)

Figure 9.4 Step-by-step guide: pleural aspiration. (a) Sterilising the area using 2% chlorhexidine in 70% isopropyl alcohol. (b) Using a blue needle to infiltrate local anaesthetic. (c) Performing a diagnostic pleural aspiration. (d) Performing a therapeutic pleural aspiration.

Cytology

- Send as much fluid as possible; aim for at least 20 mL.
- If a delay in getting the fluid to the lab is anticipated then store the sample in a fridge.

Others

- Check amylase if suspected pancreatitis.
- Check cholesterol and triglyceride if suspected chylothorax ('milky' pleural fluid).
- Check haematocrit if suspected haemothorax (present if the haematocrit of the pleural fluid is more than half of the peripheral blood haematocrit).

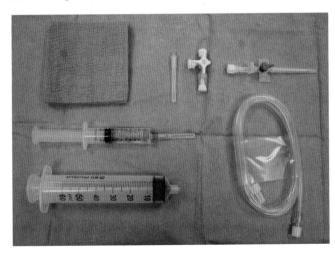

Figure 9.5 Equipment for performing therapeutic pleural aspiration.

Complications following pleural aspiration

Complications include the following.

Pneumothorax—Intercostal drain insertion may be necessary.

Bleeding—Apply direct pressure.

Spleen or liver puncture—Request an ultrasound of the chest with marking of the site for aspiration if fluid is difficult to detect.

Malignant seeding along track—If mesothelioma is suspected then mark the site of aspiration indelibly to guide radiotherapy.

Pleural effusions – clinical assessment

A pleural effusion can be defined as fluid in the pleural space. There are many causes of pleural effusions and they are commonly classified into transudates and exudates. In patients with a normal serum protein, a transudate is where the pleural fluid protein is less than 30 g/L and an exudate is where the pleural fluid protein level is greater than 30 g/L. In borderline cases (pleural fluid protein 25–35 g/L) or where the patient has an abnormal serum protein, Light's criteria can be applied. The effusion is an exudate if it meets any of the following criteria:
- pleural fluid protein : serum protein ratio >0.5
- pleural fluid LDH : serum LDH ratio >0.6
- pleural fluid LDH more than two-thirds the upper limit of normal serum LDH.

Management
Management of a patient with a pleural effusion should involve the following.
- History, examination and chest X-ray.
- Treat heart failure if present with diuretics.
- Perform pleural aspiration which may be diagnostic or therapeutic depending on the volume of fluid drained.
- Determine whether the pleural effusion is an exudate or a transudate.

Further investigations may be necessary if the diagnosis remains unclear (e.g. CT of the thorax, pleural biopsy).

Transudative pleural effusions
These are caused by either increased hydrostatic pressure or decreased osmotic pressure in the microvascular circulation. Treatment is directed at the underlying cause. Causes of transudative plural effusions can be found in Box 9.2.

Exudative pleural effusions
These are caused by an increase in capillary permeability and impaired pleural fluid reabsorption. Treatment is directed at the underlying cause as well as measures to improve symptoms and remove pleural fluid such as pleural aspiration or intercostal drain insertion. Causes of exudative pleural effusions can be found in Box 9.3.

Box 9.2 Causes of transudative pleural effusions

- Left ventricular failure
- Liver cirrhosis
- Hypoalbuminaemia
- Peritoneal dialysis
- Hypothyroidism
- Nephrotic syndrome
- Constrictive pericarditis
- Meig's syndrome (associated with ovarian tumours)

Box 9.3 Causes of exudative pleural effusions

- Malignancy
- Mesothelioma
- Parapneumonic effusions
- Empyema
- Pulmonary infarction
- Rheumatoid arthritis
- Autoimmune diseases
- Pancreatitis
- Chylothorax
- Benign asbestos effusion
- Drugs

Aspiration of a pneumothorax

A pneumothorax is defined as air in the pleural space. A primary pneumothorax can occur in healthy people with no pre-existing lung disease, whereas a secondary pneumothorax may occur in a patient with underlying lung disease (e.g. chronic obstructive pulmonary disease).

Indications for aspiration
- Primary pneumothorax if patient is symptomatic and/or a rim of air greater than 2 cm is seen on the CXR.
- Secondary pneumothorax if patient is minimally breathless, aged under 50 years of age and with a small pneumothorax (<2 cm on CXR).

Step-by-step guide: performing an aspiration of a pneumothorax
1 Give a full explanation to the patient in simple terms and ensure they agree to the procedure.
2 Set up your trolley. You will need the equipment detailed in Box 9.1 plus a three-way tap and a large cannula. You will not require the specimen containers.
3 Firstly confirm the side of the pneumothorax by clinical examination and review of the CXR.
4 A strict aseptic technique should be used.
5 The patient should be sat upright supported by pillows. The site of aspiration should be in the second intercostal space in the midclavicular line.

6 Local anaesthetic should be infiltrated into the skin, intercostal muscle and parietal pleura. Use a blue or orange needle initially followed by the green needle to infiltrate deeper. The needle should be inserted just above the upper border of the rib to avoid the intercostal neurovascular bundle. Always aspirate before injecting local anaesthetic to ensure that you are not in a blood vessel.

7 Confirm the presence of the pneumothorax by aspirating air with the green needle.

8 Whilst the local anaesthetic is left to work, attach the three-way tap to the 50-mL syringe.

9 Insert the large-bore cannula over the upper border of the rib, remove the needle and attach the three-way tap and 50-mL syringe.

10 Aspirate 50 mL of air at a time into the syringe and expel the air into the atmosphere. The patient may begin to cough during the procedure. Continue to aspirate until either resistance is felt, the patient coughs excessively, the patient experiences pain or 2.5 L of air is aspirated.

11 At the end of the procedure, remove the cannula and apply a dressing to the site.

12 Request a CXR post procedure. For a primary pneumothorax, consider a second aspiration if the first aspiration was not successful.

Learning points

- Aim to establish the cause of a pleural effusion by history, examination and pleural fluid analysis. With transudates, treatment is directed at the underlying cause, whereas with exudates, removal of the fluid with aspiration or intercostal drain insertion may be necessary.

- When performing pleural aspiration, the needle should be inserted just above the upper border of the rib to avoid the intercostal neurovascular bundle.

- If fluid is difficult to detect clinically or initial attempts at aspiration with a green (21G) needle are unsuccessful, request an ultrasound scan of the thorax with marking of a site for aspiration.

- Do not aspirate more than 1.5 L of pleural fluid due to the risk of re-expansion pulmonary oedema.

Handy hints/troubleshooting

- Always use local anaesthetic – don't be tempted to convince your patients that one needle is better than two!
- If you are suspecting that the pleural fluid might be very viscous (as with an empyema) use a large-bore needle or cannula.
- Remember to prescribe some PRN post-procedure analgesia.
- Always monitor the patient throughout the procedure; the pulse oximeter is particularly important.

Further reading

Antunes G, Neville E, Duffy J, Ali N. (2003) BTS Guidelines for the Management of Malignant Pleural Effusions. *Thorax* 58 (Suppl II): ii29–ii38.

Chapman S, Robinson G, Stradling J, West S. (2005) *Oxford Handbook of Respiratory Medicine*. Oxford University Press, Oxford.

Davies CWH, Gleeson FV, Davies RJO. (2003) BTS Guidelines for the Management of Pleural Infection. *Thorax* 58 (Suppl II): ii18–ii28.

Henry M, Arnold T, Harvey J. (2003) BTS Guidelines for the Management of Spontaneous Pneumothorax. *Thorax* 58 (Suppl II): ii39–ii52.

Light RW. (2002) Pleural effusion. *N Engl J Med* 346 (25); 1971–7.

Maskell NA, Butland RJA. (2003) BTS Guidelines for the Investigation of a Unilateral Pleural Effusion in Adults. *Thorax* 58 (suppl II); ii8–ii17.

CHAPTER 10

Access: Intravenous Cannulation

Anna Fergusson[1] and Oliver Masters[2]

[1]*Russells Hall Hospital, Dudley, UK*
[2]*Queen Elizabeth Hospital, Birmingham, UK*

OVERVIEW

By the end of this chapter you should be able to:
- discuss the indications and contraindications for peripheral cannulation
- understand the anatomy of potential cannulation sites
- identify the correct site and size for a cannula
- understand the potential complications of peripheral cannulation
- describe the technique for insertion of a cannula.

Introduction

Peripheral venous cannulation is one of the most common invasive procedures carried out in hospital. Thousands of cannulae are inserted every day in the UK, mostly by junior doctors or nurses. Peripheral venous cannulation is associated with significant morbidity and mortality – mainly secondary to infection. It has been estimated that an episode of bacteraemia occurs for 1 in every 100 peripheral cannulae sited. It is therefore essential not only to be capable of competently putting in a cannula correctly, but also to do this in a safe manner.

Before inserting a cannula it is essential to determine whether or not there is a clinical indication. Studies show that up to one third of cannulae in hospitalised patients are not required or are not being used. Alternatives to cannulation should be considered where possible; for example oral antibiotics instead of intravenous antibiotics, or encouragement of oral fluid intake instead of intravenous fluids.

Indications

- Intravenous fluids.
- Intravenous drugs – continuous or intermittent.
- Blood or blood products.
- Intravenous radio-opaque contrast or sedation.
- Prophylactic use in unstable patients or those undergoing procedures.

ABC of Practical Procedures. Edited by T. Nutbeam and R. Daniels. © 2010
Blackwell Publishing, ISBN: 978-1-4051-8595-0.

Contraindications

Absolute

- Inflammation or infection of overlying skin at proposed cannula site.
- Arteriovenous (AV) fistula in arm of proposed cannula site.
- Previous mastectomy with axillary node surgery or lymphoedema on side of proposed upper limb cannulation.

Relative

- Bleeding tendency.
- Veins of the forearm (elbow to wrist) in those with renal failure who may require AV fistula formation in the future.

Anatomy of veins

Veins consist of three layers: the tunica adventitia, tunica media, and tunica intima. Veins contain valves, folds of endothelium, which assist with flow of blood back to the heart. Valves can sometimes be identified by palpation of small bulges in the vein. Figure 10.1 shows the anatomy of the veins of the hand.

Cannulae

A cannula is composed of several parts: the needle, catheter, wings, valve, injection port and Luer-Lok™ cap. Most cannulae also contain a 'flashback chamber' giving the practitioner visual confirmation that the cannula has entered the vein. Figure 10.2 shows a labelled diagram of a cannula.

Modern peripheral cannulae are made from polyurethane. This is preferable to older materials such as PVC and Teflon® as the cannulae are more flexible, softer and cause less intimal damage. They are also latex free.

Table 10.1 shows sizes of cannulae, colour, flow rates and uses. Remember that the maximum flow rate is printed on the packaging of most cannulae – important if you are fluid resuscitating!

Choosing the appropriate cannula

Deciding on the appropriate-sized cannula and the appropriate vein will depend on a number of factors. In a resuscitation situation, or if the patient is unstable, the biggest cannula that the

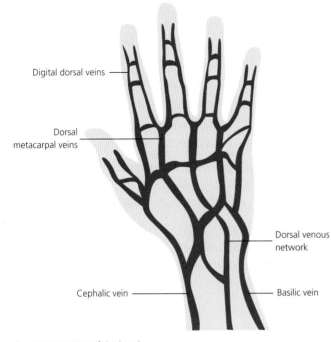

Figure 10.1 Veins of the hand.

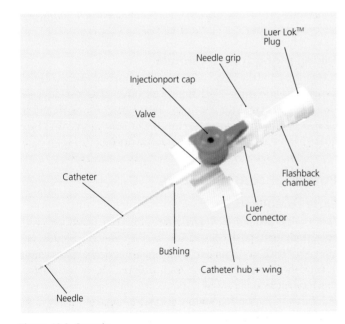

Figure 10.2 Cannula.

practitioner is competent to insert should be put into the patient's largest peripheral vein. This will usually be a 14G or 16G (orange or grey) cannula in the antecubital fossa. These cannulae have the largest radius and therefore the highest flow rate, allowing a large volume of fluid to enter the circulating volume in a short period of time. By doubling the radius of the cannula, the flow through it is increased 16-fold.

A cannula inserted into a large vein is needed in situations where potentially irritant drugs need to be administered and the insertion

Table 10.1 Cannula sizes and their uses.

Colour	Size	Flow rate		Use
Blue	22G	36 mL/min	2.2L/h	Paediatric or elderly patients with small, fragile veins
Pink	20G	61 mL/min	3.7L/h	IV maintenance fluids, drugs,
Green	18G	90 mL/min	5.4L/h	blood products
White	17G	140 mL/min	6.2L/h	Rapid infusions of fluids, drugs
Grey	16G	200 mL/min	12L/h	and blood products.
Brown/ orange	14G	300 mL/min	18L/h	Unstable patients, emergency situations

of a central line is not appropriate. Examples of such drugs include 50% glucose for the treatment of hypoglycaemia and amiodarone for arrhythmias.

An 18G or 20G (green or pink) cannula is appropriate for situations where maintenance fluid or IV drugs are required. 22G (blue) cannulae should be reserved for children or those with very difficult IV access. Blood products should be run through a 18G (green) or bigger cannula to minimise the risk of clotting.

Choosing the site of cannulation

Choosing the ideal vein for cannulation should take into consideration factors such as patient comfort and convenience, size of cannula required, and the size, mobility and fragility of the patient's veins. Where possible, the patient's non-dominant hand should be chosen. The back of the hand or lower arm should be chosen in most situations, as it is relatively comfortable, the cannula is unlikely to kink and it is easily inspected and accessed. Cannulation of the hand is also associated with a lower incidence of phlebitis compared with cannulation of veins of the wrist or upper arm. The distal cephalic vein, known as the 'houseman`s vein' because it is often chosen by junior doctors, is normally large and well tethered, making it easy to cannulate. Veins in the antecubital fossa are often large and easy to cannulate, but can be awkward and obstruction of flow through the cannula tends to occur if the elbow is flexed.

Veins on the underside of the arm and wrist are often painful when cannulated so should be avoided if possible. Veins in the foot can be used as a last resort but tend to be painful and inconvenient for the patient and are associated with a higher risk of phlebitis and thromboembolism. Finally, experienced practitioners will occasionally cannulate the external jugular vein, particularly in emergency situations when IV access elsewhere is difficult.

Step-by-step guide: intravenous cannulation

- **Give a full explanation to the patient in simple terms and ensure they consent to the procedure (if able).**
- **Set up your trolley (Box 10.1 and Figure 10.3).**
- **Prepare your trolley as a sterile field. Wear a plastic disposable apron and non-sterile gloves, and take alcohol hand rub with you.**

Box 10.1 **Equipment for intravenous cannulation**

- Gloves
- Tourniquet (disposable if available)
- 2% chlorhexidine/alcohol wipe
- Cannula
- Gauze
- Sharps bin
- 5 mL 0.9% saline
- 5-mL syringe
- Cannula dressing

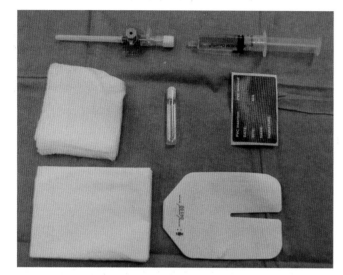

Figure 10.3 Equipment required for intravenous cannulation.

1 Position the patient comfortably. It may be helpful to have the arm resting on a pillow.
2 Apply the tourniquet to the upper arm (Figure 10.4a). It should not be so tight as to obstruct arterial blood flow – check by palpating the radial pulse.
3 Ask the patient to clench and unclench the fist. This will promote venous filling.
4 Look and palpate for appropriate veins; they should feel full and bouncy. The site of a vein bifurcation is often ideal as the vein is tethered at this point.
5 Clean the area with an appropriate product: 2% chlorhexidine gluconate in 70% isopropyl alcohol is recommended (Figure 10.4b). Remember to let the solution dry and not to palpate the skin further (no-touch technique).
6 Remove the cap from the cannula and put in a clean, safe, easily accessible place (alternatively the cap can be left in place and removed at the end of the procedure).
7 Hold the skin taut below your insertion site to tether and immobilise the vein.
8 Holding the cannula at a 10–30º angle to the skin and in the direction of the vein, gently advance the cannula through the skin and into the vein (Figure 10.4c).
9 Once a flashback has been seen in the flashback chamber (Figure 10.4d), lower the cannula slightly to ensure the tip is in the lumen of the vein and that the needle does not puncture the posterior wall of the vein, then advance the cannula a further few millimetres. Figure 10.5 shows a diagrammatic representation of this.
10 Withdraw the needle gently and watch for the second flashback in the cannula confirming that it is in the correct position (Figure 10.4e).
11 Slowly advance the cannula fully into the vein holding the wings of the cannula only (Figure 10.4f).
12 Remove the tourniquet.
13 Place a small piece of gauze underneath the open end of the cannula to catch any drops of blood (Figure 10.4g).
14 Occlude the vein proximal to the tip of the cannula with your finger while removing the needle from the cannula (Figure 10.4h).
15 Dispose of the sharp safely before screwing the cap securely on the end of the cannula.
16 Secure the cannula safely with a purpose-made, sterile, semi-permeable transparent dressing (Figure 10.4i).
17 If the dressing allows, label it with the insertion date and time.
18 Flush the cannula via the injection port with 5 mL 0.9% saline (Figure 10.4j). Observe for any swelling or pain proximal to the cannula site which could indicate that the cannula is not correctly positioned.
19 Document the procedure, including the date and time, size of cannula used, site, number of attempts, and any immediate complications.

Taking blood from a cannula

It is possible to take blood out of a newly inserted cannula before the cannula is flushed. This is done with either a purpose-designed Vacutainer™ adapter or a syringe (Figure 10.6). Blood should be taken before the tourniquet is released. Once the cannula has been flushed, it should not be used for blood sampling.

Potential complications

Early complications

Early complications of cannulation are often associated with poor technique and inexperienced practitioners. If the primary flashback does not occur, the vein has probably not been punctured. Re-palpate the vein and withdraw the cannula before re-advancing again. If this is unsuccessful, start again and choose a different site. For tips on finding a suitable vein, see 'Handy hints' box below.

If the secondary flashback (as the needle is withdrawn through the cannula) does not occur, the cannula is no longer in the vein. This may be because the cannula entered the vein and then passed through the posterior wall. By slowly withdrawing you may then get a flashback as it re-enters the vein, in which case you can carefully advance the cannula into the vein. Once the needle has been withdrawn it should not be re-inserted into the cannula. This practice may cause part of the catheter to be sheared off by the needle, therefore entering the systemic circulation.

Cannulation is often a relatively painful experience for the patient. This is more of a problem when larger cannulae are being used or when cannulating children. In these circumstances subcutaneous or topical local anaesthetic can be used.

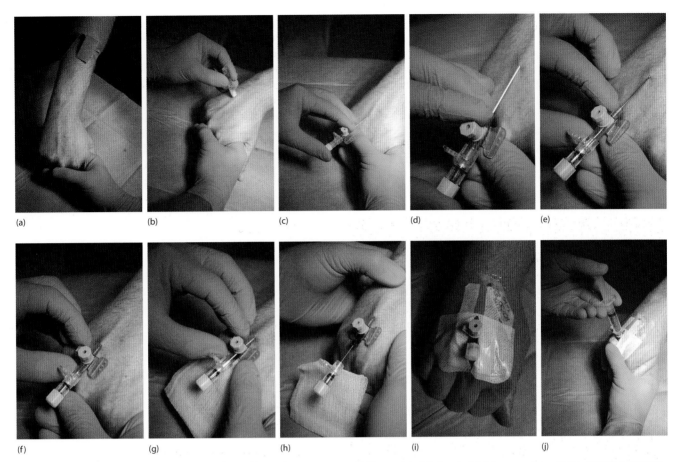

(a) (b) (c) (d) (e)

(f) (g) (h) (i) (j)

Figure 10.4 Step-by-step guide: intravenous cannulation. (a) Tourniquet on the forearm. (b) Sterilising the insertion site with 2% chlorhexidine gluconate in 70% isopropyl alcohol. (c) The insertion angle of 10–30°. (d) The first flashback seen in the hub of the cannula. (e) Secondary flashback in the cannula itself.

(f) The cannula fully inserted. (g) Gauze underneath the cannula to prevent blood spillage. (h) Removing the needle from the cannula. (i) The cannula fully dressed and dated (the insertion point can be easily observed through the dressing). (j) The cannula is flushed with 0.9% saline.

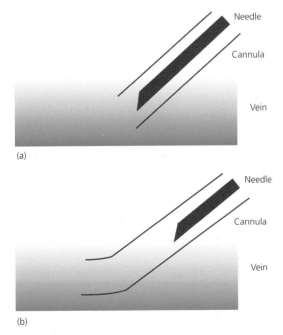

(a)

(b)

Figure 10.5 Diagrammatic representation of cannulation. (a) The needle and cannula enter the lumen of the vein. The primary flashback is seen. (b) The needle is withdrawn and the cannula advanced into the lumen. The secondary flashback is seen.

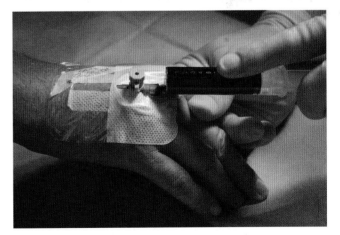

Figure 10.6 Taking blood out of a cannula. Blood is withdrawn from the cannula using a 10-mL syringe.

Haematoma formation is a common complication of cannulation. A collection of blood forms in the soft tissue following leakage of blood from a venous puncture site. Haematoma is a common feature of failed cannulation or accidentally displaced cannulae. It is often more severe in those who are anticoagulated or have deranged clotting. The cannula must be removed and pressure applied to the area for at least 3 minutes to reduce bruising.

Occasionally it is possible to 'hit a valve'. This may manifest in difficulty threading the cannula up the vein. Careful palpation of the vein to locate the valves may help avoid this problem; valves can be felt as small bulges. It may also be possible to advance the cannula while flushing it with normal saline. This may cause the valve to open to allow the cannula through.

Rarely, an artery can be cannulated accidentally. This may have catastrophic consequences if unrecognised and the cannula is used to administer drugs. It is more likely to occur when cannulating veins in the antecubital fossa or the cephalic vein. At these sites either the brachial artery or an anatomical variant of the radial artery may be cannulated. Arterial cannulation is more likely in overweight patients, where the veins are very deep and difficult to palpate, or in very thin patients. It is usually obvious as the blood is redder than expected and pulsatile. If there is any doubt the cannula should be removed immediately and pressure applied for at least 5 minutes.

Needlestick injuries can occur when cannulating. Self-blunting or retractable cannula are available, minimising the risk of needlestick injuries, and should be used where possible. For further information on needlestick injuries refer to Chapter 3.

Late complications

Phlebitis is inflammation of the vein and can be due to chemical or mechanical irritation, or infection. Thrombophlebitis occurs when phlebitis is associated with formation of a thrombus within the vessel. Phlebitis and thrombophlebitis are extremely common, occurring in up to 35% of cannulations. They present with erythema, swelling, warmth, tenderness, and occasionally a palpable venous cord. Risk factors include the length of time the cannula is in situ, infusion of irritant drugs or fluids, and which material the cannula is manufactured from.

The vast majority of infective phlebitis is superficial and requires no treatment other than removal of the cannula. Oral antibiotics may be considered. Occasionally, systemic sepsis can occur, with an incidence of 1 per 3000 peripheral cannulae in one large study. Between 1997 and 2002, 6.2% of hospital-acquired bacteraemias were caused by peripheral IV cannulae.

Contamination can occur when skin flora is introduced at cannula insertion or by the introduction of other organisms via the cannula hub or injection port. The commonest organisms responsible for infective phlebitis are coagulase-negative staphylococcus and *Staphylococcus aureus* (40–45% of which are methicillin-resistant *Staphylococcus aureus*).

The risk of cannula site infection can be minimised by using an aseptic technique (particularly important in patients who are immunosuppressed), regular inspection, and minimal time in situ (no cannula should be left in situ for more than 72 hours). A high index of suspicion is vital in any patient with a cannula in situ who becomes septic with no obvious cause. Finally, it is important to assess each patient's clinical indication and avoid cannulation where possible.

Thromboembolism can occur, where blood clots on the cannula or vein wall before breaking off and being carried into the heart and pulmonary circulation. There is also a small risk of air embolism, especially if care is not taken to prime all administration equipment appropriately.

Extravasation, or 'tissueing', is a common problem, occurring in up to a quarter of those receiving intravenous infusions. This occurs when infusion fluid or drug leaks into the subcutaneous tissues surrounding the vein, normally when the cannula is dislodged from the vein or the tip is sitting in the vessel wall. Extravasation presents with localised pain and swelling. Careful monitoring of the cannula site is needed, especially in those who cannot communicate efficiently, such as children, the elderly or those with reduced consciousness.

Care of cannula site

Once inserted, the cannula should be secured appropriately, using a purpose-made adhesive dressing. This should be transparent around the cannula site to allow direct inspection when looking for any signs of phlebitis. It may be necessary to apply a loose-fitting bandage over the cannula to increase its security, especially in a confused or agitated patient. In this case it is vital that the bandage is regularly removed to actively look for any evidence of phlebitis.

The cannula site should be inspected every 8 hours as a minimum, and a phlebitis scale used, such as the Visual Infusion Phlebitis score (VIP score – see Table 10.2). If phlebitis is noted, this

Table 10.2 Visual Infusion Phlebitis (VIP) score. Developed by Andrew Jackson, Consultant Nurse Intravenous Therapy and Care, Rotherham General Hospitals NHS Trust.

0	IV site appears healthy	No signs of phlebitis • Observe cannula
1	One of the following is evident: • Slight pain near IV site • Slight redness near IV site	Possible signs of phlebitis • Observe cannula
2	Two of the following are evident: • Pain near IV site • Erythema • Swelling	Early stages of phlebitis • Resite cannula
3	All of the following are evident: • Pain along path of cannula • Erythema • Induration	Medium stage of phlebitis • Resite cannula • Consider treatment
4	All of the following are evident and extensive: • Pain along path of cannula • Erythema • Induration • Palpable venous cord	Advanced stages of phlebitis or start of thrombophlebitis • Resite cannula • Consider treatment
5	All of the following and evident and extensive: • Pain along path of cannula • Erythema • Induration • Palpable venous cord • Pyrexia	Advanced stage of thrombophlebitis • Initiate treatment • Resite cannula

should be documented, and the cannula either removed or closely observed (in cases of mild phlebitis). A doctor's opinion should be sought and antibiotics considered if infection is present.

All cannulae should be removed after 72 hours, regardless or whether or not they look infected. The risk of infection rises rapidly with time beyond this. Cannulae no longer in use should be removed as soon as possible to prevent complications.

Summary

Intravenous cannulation is a very common, simple procedure and makes up a large part of the 'bread and butter' work for most junior doctors. However, it is often a life-saving procedure and can occasionally be very challenging. Venous cannulation is associated with a number of complications, resulting in considerable morbidity, prolonged hospitalisation and even death. It is vital that healthcare practitioners are competent at cannulation, including cannulation in emergency situations, and that you are aware of the potential problems and how to manage them.

Handy hints/troubleshooting

- Always have a good look at both hands before deciding on the best vein.
- Veins in the antecubital fossa are often easiest (but more uncomfortable for the patient and the cannula will often kink).
- Make sure the area is as well lit as possible, even in the middle of the night.
- Remember, a good vein is one you can feel but not always see!
- Ask the patient to hang his or her hand down and to clench and release the hand.
- Tapping the vein gently will vasodilate the vein and make it stand out.
- If you're really struggling, try putting the hands in warm water or applying a GTN patch – both act as vasodilators, giving you a bigger target!

Further reading

Centers for Disease Control and Prevention. (2002) *Guidelines for the Prevention of Intravascular Catheter-related Infections.* MMWR Recommendations and Reports 51, RR-10, 1–29.

Department of Health. (2007) *High Impact Intervention No 2. Peripheral Intravenous Cannula Care Bundle.* www.dh.gov.uk/en/Publichealth/Healthprotection/Healthcareacquiredinfection/Healthcareacquiredgeneralinformation/ThedeliveryprogrammetoreducehealthcareassociatedinfectionsHCAI includingMRSA/index.htm

Department of Health. (2003) *Winning ways: Working Together to Reduce Associated Healthcare Infection in England.* www.dh.gov.uk/en/Publicationsandstatistics/Publications/PublicationsPolicyAndGuidance/Browsable/DH_4095070

Dougherty L, Lister S. (2008) *The Royal Marsden NHS Trust Manual of Clinical Nursing Procedures,* 7th edn. Wiley-Blackwell, Oxford.

Nosocomial Infection National Surveillance Service (NINSS). (2002) *Surveillance of Hospital Acquired Bacteraemia in English Hospital 1997–2002. A National Surveillance and Quality Improvement Program.* www.hpa.org.uk/infections/publications/ninns/hosacq_HAB_2002.pdf

CHAPTER 11

Access: Central Venous

Ronan O'Leary[1] and Andrew Quinn[2]

[1]*Yorkshire Deanery, York, UK*
[2]*Department of Anaesthesia, Bradford Royal Infirmary, Bradford, UK*

OVERVIEW

By the end of this chapter you should be able to:

- explain both the benefits and risks of central venous access
- understand the anatomy of the internal jugular, subclavian and femoral veins
- explain both anatomical landmark and ultrasound-guided techniques for central line insertion
- understand the potential complications of this invasive procedure.

Introduction

Central venous access is a frequently performed invasive procedure which carries a significant risk of morbidity and even mortality. It is usual for this procedure to be carried out in operating theatre or high-dependency care areas, always using a fully aseptic technique. Ultrasound can be used to identify the vessels and to avoid important nearby structures.

Central venous access refers to lines placed into the large veins of the neck, chest, or groin. To measure central venous pressure, the tip must lie within the thoracic cavity and preferably in the superior vena cava. As such, the femoral route is suboptimal for this purpose. The device may be inserted directly into a central vein, tunnelled subcutaneously and then inserted into a central vein or inserted via a peripheral vein.

Indications

- Monitoring (these techniques are discussed in more detail in Chapter 19).
- Infusion of irritant drugs that may damage smaller veins.
- Insertion of pacing wires.
- Renal replacement therapy.
- Emergency venous access.
- Parenteral feeding.
- Resuscitation of patients who are intravascularly depleted.

ABC of Practical Procedures. Edited by T. Nutbeam and R. Daniels. © 2010 Blackwell Publishing, ISBN: 978-1-4051-8595-0.

Contraindications

Given the wide range of indications for central venous access it is difficult to describe any absolute contraindications other than patient refusal. Relative contraindications depend on the clinical indication, the skill and experience of the operator, and where the patient will be nursed after insertion. The most important relative contraindications:

- uncorrected coagulopathy
- thrombocytopenia
- skin infection over the site of access
- obscure anatomical landmarks
- haemo- or pneumothorax on the contralateral side
- recent surgery to other structures nearby such as carotid endartectomy.

Rare contraindications include arteriovenous malformations, renal cell tumour extension into the right atrium, and fungating tricuspid valve vegetations.

Anatomy

It is impossible to understate the importance of knowing the anatomy relevant to central venous access. A good way to learn these techniques is to position a colleague in the manner described in these sections and to identify the landmarks, vessels and pulsations.

Internal jugular vein (IJV)

The IJV runs from its origin at the jugular foramen to the sternal margin of the clavicle. Here it terminates by joining the subclavian vein (SCV) to form the brachiocephalic vein (Figure 11.1).

The IJV is surrounded by the carotid sheath which also contains the carotid artery, and the vagus nerve. When the vein forms it initially lies very superficially in the anterior triangle of the neck and overlies the internal carotid artery. As it descends it moves to lie laterally to the artery.

Subclavian vein (SCV)

The SCV is a continuation of the axillary vein. It begins at the outer border of the first rib and ends at the medial border of scalenus anterior, where it joins the internal jugular vein to form the brachiocephalic vein behind the sternoclavicular joint.

Femoral vein

The femoral vein is the continuation of the popliteal vein and ends medial to the artery at the inguinal ligament where it becomes the external iliac vein. The femoral artery, vein and nerve lie within the femoral triangle, arranged from lateral to medial: nerve, artery, vein (Figure 11.2). The artery can easily be palpated on a subject, and the vein lies 2 cm medial to the pulsation.

Site selection

The anatomy of these areas is complex and the risk of damaging nearby structures is significant. The choice of site depends on a combination of factors, which are summarised in Table 11.1.

Ultrasound

The use of ultrasound scanning (USS) has significantly reduced the complications from central venous access. Two-dimensional ultrasound can be employed to identify the relevant veins and accompanying artery and can be used throughout the procedure to confirm venous cannulation and finally at the end of the procedure to confirm catheter placement in the vein. USS may also demonstrate thrombosis, stenosis and anatomical variants that may preclude catheter insertion. Given the relatively low cost of USS equipment and the straightforward training required to perform USS-guided central venous access it has become the standard technique for elective line placement.

The step-by-step guide in this chapter covers insertion techniques with and without ultrasound. It is important to learn both, as the landmark technique is invaluable in emergency situations.

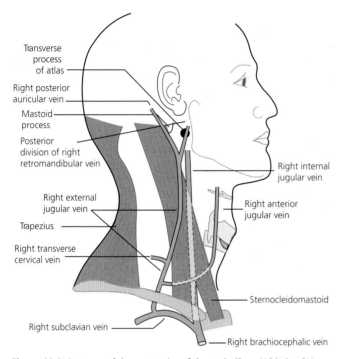

Figure 11.1 Anatomy of the great veins of the neck. (From Whitaker RH, Borley NR. (2005) *Instant Anatomy*, 3rd edn. Blackwell Publishing, Oxford, with permission.)

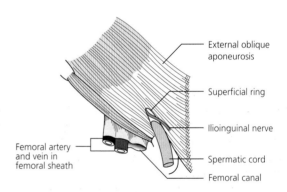

Figure 11.2 Anatomy of the femoral artery. (From Faiz O, Moffat D. (2006) *Anatomy at a Glance*, 2nd edn. Blackwell Publishing, Oxford, with permission.)

Table 11.1 Factors to consider when choosing a site for central venous access.

Site	Advantages	Potential for complications	Other factors
Internal jugular	Anatomy readily visible with ultrasound Can be adapted to accommodate patient size and position Easily accessed surface of patient	Puncture of internal carotid or misplaced line in the internal carotid Pneumothorax is a recognised complication	Difficult to nurse long term Dressings can be problematic due to beard/stubble Uncomfortable for patient
Subclavian	Lower risk of infection Does not require movement of patient's head and can be accessed during c-spine immobilisation Useful in emergencies Vein does not collapse fully in hypovolaemic states	Highest chance of pneumothorax Puncture of tracheostomy or endotracheal tube cuff Cannot apply pressure to stop bleeding Can be painful even with good skin anaesthesia Less easy to visualise with USS	Easier to nurse Comfortable for patient
Femoral	Safest vein to place large lines, for example for veno–veno haemofiltration because there are fewer important structures nearby. Puncture of femoral artery can usually be treated with pressure	Femoral artery puncture leading to retroperitoneal bleed Femoral nerve damage Difficult to nurse and keep clean Highest likelihood of infection	Patient position is comfortable for the patient Easy to anaesthetise all tissues which will be punctured, cut or dilated

Step-by-step guide: right internal jugular central venous access

> • Give a full explanation to the patient in simple terms and ensure they consent to the procedure (if able).
> • Set up your trolley (Box 11.1 and Figure 11.3).
> • Ensure the pressurised monitoring system is set up.
> • Prepare your trolley as a sterile field. Wear a plastic disposable apron and non-sterile gloves, and take alcohol hand rub with you.

1 After setting up the trolley, discard gloves and apron used, re-wash hands and don a new pair of non-sterile gloves and apron.
2 Before putting on sterile gloves, position the patient. The patient should be on a trolley which can be tipped head down (Trendelenberg position) and the area should be exposed, whilst maintaining as much dignity as possible. Positioning the patient correctly is the key to success (Box 11.2). A head-down position should be used when cannulating to minimise the risk of venous air embolism.
3 Scrub and wear a sterile gown, gloves and a facemask. Consider eye protection. You will need an assistant to help to finalise your preparations, talk to the patient and go for help should problems arise.
4 Ask your assistant to pour saline into your Gallipot. Attach three-way taps to all but the central lumen and flush each line with saline. Turn the taps to the closed position. Place the line back onto the draped trolley.
5 Clean the skin with antiseptic (2% chlorhexidine in 70% isopropyl alcohol is recommended) and drape the area (Figure 11.4a,b). A sterile technique should be maintained throughout insertion and securing the central line.

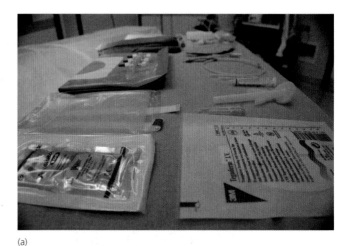

(a)

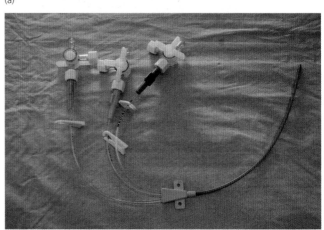

(b)

Figure 11.3 Equipment required for central venous cannulation. (a) Correctly prepared trolley, which includes the components of a commercially available central line kit, drapes, cleaning solution, ultrasound probe cover and dressings. (b) A typical three-lumen central line with three-way taps attached.

Box 11.1 **Equipment for central venous cannulation**

Central line kit containing:
• needle or a cannula over needle
• central venous catheter
• guidewire
• dilator
• anchoring clips.

Additional items:
• suture
• scalpel
• appropriate dressing
• syringes
• blue and green needles
• three-way taps, one for each lumen
• drapes
• cleaning fluid (2% chlorhexidine gluconate in 70% isopropyl alcohol is recommended)
• swabs
• Gallipot or similar
• sterile ultrasound probe sheath
• 0.9% normal saline.

Box 11.2 **Patient positioning**

Internal jugular
The patient should be lying as flat as possible with the head resting on one pillow and turned to look to the contralateral side. The trolley should be tipped head down to about 15°, the Trendelenburg position, which distends the veins and decreases the risk of air embolism. Place a large absorbent pad under the patient's head and shoulders to protect the bedclothes from cleaning fluid and blood.

Subclavian
As for IJ except that a pillow should be placed under the upper back and the head allowed to fall backwards onto the bed rather than onto the pillow.

Femoral
Place the patient flat, and abduct the leg to about 30°, or even let the leg hang over the side of the bed.
    Identify the femoral artery and vein and ensure that an imaginary line passing through the femoral vein to the iliac veins and onto the inferior vena cava is approximately straight.

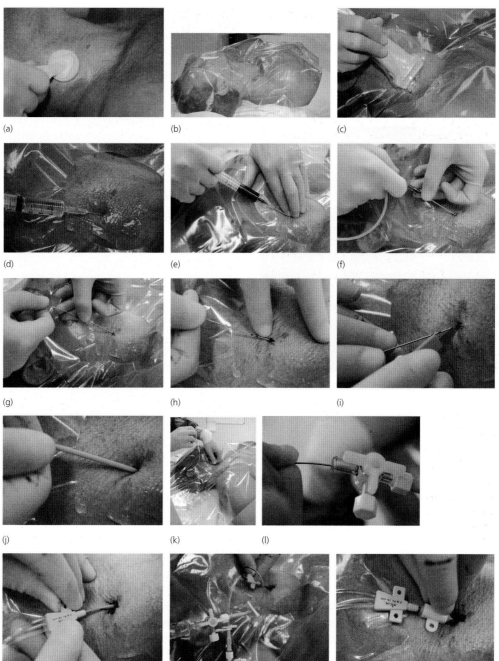

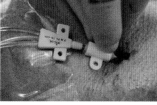

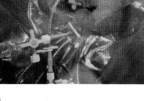

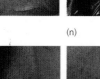

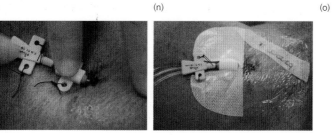

Figure 11.4 Step-by-step guide: central venous access. (a) Sterilising insertion site with a commercially available preparation of 2% chlorhexidine gluconate in 70% isopropyl alcohol. (b) Patient draped with 'aperture' sterile drape. (c) Using a draped US probe to identify insertion landmarks. (d) Infiltrating local anaesthetic (1% lidocaine) around identified insertion site. (e) Aspirating blood from internal jugular. (f) Using wire introducer. (g) Guidewire inserted through needle. (h) Guidewire in situ. (i) Cutting down onto wire with scalpel. (j) Dilating over guidewire. (k) Inserting central line over guidewire. (l) Ensuring guidewire is securely held as central line is introduced. (m) Line inserted to 15 cm depth. (n) Aspirating all ports of line (flashback can be clearly seen). (o) Placing secure clips over wire. (p) Clips sutured into position to secure wire. (q) Line dressed clearly showing insertion site.

Box 11.3 **Use of US probe**

The vein will usually be larger and lateral to the artery which will have a visible arterial pulsation. Compress the neck with the probe; the vein should be compressible and the artery will retain its shape.

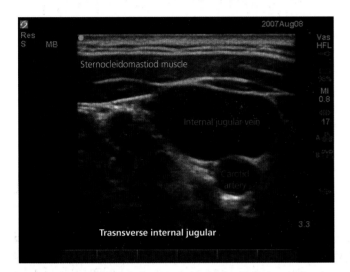

Figure 11.5 An ultrasound view showing the landmarks for internal jugular cannulation.

6 If using ultrasound the probe should be covered with a sterile cover (Figure 11.4c). Single-use sterile ultrasound transmission gel should be applied to provide contact between the probe and the plastic cover and also between the sheath and the patient.

7 Identify the site of skin puncture. Local anaesthetic (e.g. 1% lidocaine) should be infiltrated around this site (Figure 11.4d).

8 The ultrasound probe can now be placed over the anaesthetised area and the vein and artery can be visualised (Box 11.3 and Figure 11.5).

9 Move the probe up and down the neck slightly to find the position where the vein is largest and most lateral to the artery (or use the landmark techniques described in Box 11.4).

10 Use the introducer needle attached to a 10-mL syringe, approaching the skin at a 30° angle. Begin to aspirate as soon as you pierce the skin (Figure 11.4e). If using USS insert the needle just proximal to the probe and watch the screen at all times. The needle will appear as a bright white, echo-dense, spot which you can angle towards the vein until it deforms the wall of the vein as it pierces it.

11 As soon as blood is aspirated stop advancing the needle. USS can be used to confirm the location of the needle in the vein.

12 Remove the syringe, and keep hold of the needle; the blood should flow gently rather than with a pulsatile spurt (this suggests arterial puncture).

13 The guidewire should be inserted into the introducer needle (Figure 11.4f,g). It should pass freely without resistance. During insertion of the guidewire the ECG should be observed. If the

Box 11.4 **Surface landmarks for needle insertion**

Right internal jugular vein

Identify the sternocleidomastoid and look for where the sternal and clavicular heads divide. The IJV runs directly beneath the apex formed by the bifurcation of the two muscle bellies. The internal carotid artery is palpated and gently lifted medially. The vein now lies lateral to the artery.

In a healthy well-hydrated subject lying on a trolley tipped head down, the IJV pulsation may be visible and the vein fills and empties.

The JVP waveform is different to the carotid pulsation because it is more complex, present in diastole, of lower amplitude and non-palpable.

Insert the needle at 30° to the skin aiming for the ipsilateral nipple as shown in the step-by-step guide. The vein lies less than 1 cm below the skin in a slim subject.

Right subclavian vein

Neither the subclavian artery or vein can be directly visualised or palpated. The key surface landmark is the clavicle. Palpate it along its entire length and establish the point between the medial third and the middle third. This lies on the most curved part of the clavicle where it turns to run posteriorly.

The needle is introduced at this point and passed under the clavicle. It is essential to keep a mental image of where the tip of the needle lies. When it is under the clavicle, flatten the syringe to the skin and aim for the suprasternal notch. The SCV should be reached at approximately 4 cm.

Right femoral vein

Identify the femoral triangle at the top of the thigh below the inguinal ligament. To do this find the pubic tubercle and palpate laterally until the femoral artery pulsation is felt. The vein lies 2 cm medial to the femoral artery. Approach the skin one finger's breadth medial to the artery at 30° aiming for the contralateral shoulder.

guidewire passes too far and touches the endocardium, atrial or ventricular ectopics can be observed. If this occurs withdraw the wire immediately.

14 When the guidewire has been inserted to an appropriate length (look for marker) the needle can be withdrawn (Figure 11.4h).

15 *It is essential that one hand keeps hold of the guidewire throughout the rest of the procedure, until the wire is removed.*

16 If using USS place the probe over the vein, the guidewire will be visible in the vein lumen.

17 Use a scalpel to make a small nick in the skin around the insertion point of the guidewire (Figure 11.4i).

18 Pass the dilator over the wire and dilate the skin and subcutaneous tissue only, keeping hold of the wire at all times (Figure 11.4j).

19 Remove the dilator while holding a sterile swab over the insertion site. Place the central line over the wire and pass the line into the vein (Figure 11.4k,l).

20 Stop advancing the cannula at a depth of 15 cm and remove the wire, keeping hold of the central line (Figure 11.4m).

21 Use a syringe filled with saline to check that you can aspirate blood from each lumen and that they each flush freely (Figure 11.4n).

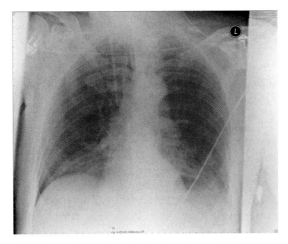

Figure 11.6 A correctly positioned central line (IJ approach).

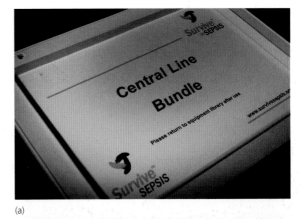

(a)

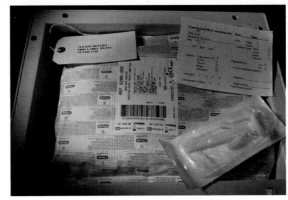

(b)

Figure 11.7 Central line care bundle. (a) Box. (b) Box contents.

> Box 11.5 **Central line care bundle**
>
> The key components of the central line bundle are:
> - hand hygiene
> - maximal barrier precautions upon insertion
> - chlorhexidine skin antisepsis
> - optimal catheter site selection, with subclavian vein as the preferred site for non-tunnelled catheters
> - avoid the femoral site unless it is the last resort
> - daily review of line with prompt removal of unnecessary lines.

22 Remove the syringe, turn the three-way tap off and cap the line. When flushing the distal line, a three-way tap needs to be attached first.

23 The line should then be attached to the skin using a suture and the locking clips (Figure 11.4o,p). The distal portion of many lines also has loops for suturing so that the line is attached at four points. Finally, clean and dry the site. Dress the area with transparent semipermeable dressing (Figure 11.4q).

24 Order a chest X-ray to check tip position; in the superior vena cava above the pericardial reflection, and to check for complications (Figure 11.6).

Postinsertion care

Central lines are a frequent site of colonisation by microorganisms that can cause catheter-related bloodstream infections. Strict attention is paid to the prevention and recognition of infection around lines. Central line care bundles have been developed to minimise this risk; an example is shown in Box 11.5 and Figure 11.7.

Complications

There are several potentially serious complications to be aware of when inserting central venous catheters.

Table 11.1 describes the common complications of the internal jugular, subclavian and femoral approaches.

All forms of venous access, but especially central access, may cause air embolism which can have catastrophic consequences. This occurs when air is aspirated into the vein during the procedure. The air embolus can translocate to the lung and if the volume is sufficient it can cause fatal cardiovascular and respiratory collapse. The likelihood may be reduced by keeping the patient in a head-down position and ensuring that the vein is open to the external environment for as little time as possible.

The carotid or subclavian artery may be either punctured or cannulated which may cause stroke, haemorrhage, and inadvertent administration of drugs into the arterial system. Good technique should reduce the possibility of inadvertent arterial cannulation; furthermore USS-guided placement is likely to increase success. Subsequently if the central line is transduced (see Chapter 19) a central venous, rather than arterial, waveform should be observed.

Other techniques to confirm cannulation of the correct vessel include transducing the needle before passing the guidewire or using a blood gas machine to analyse the blood from the vessel for oxygen content.

Less common complications include chylothorax, vagus nerve damage (IJV), and puncture of the myocardium leading to pericardial tamponade. Venous thrombosis is a potential complication for all of the veins discussed here, especially the femoral.

If the guidewire is lost within the patient (Figure 11.8) then interventional radiologists, or vascular or cardiac surgeons

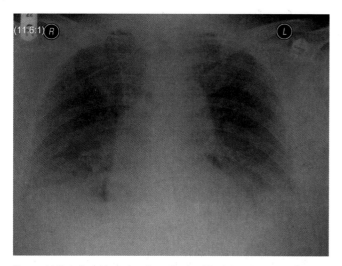

Figure 11.8 A chest X-ray showing a 'lost' guidewire: an emergent thoracic opinion is indicated.

Handy hints/troubleshooting

- The most common complication of this procedure is infection; strict aseptic technique must be adhered to.
- Always spend time positioning your patient; this maximises the chances of success first pass.
- Read the notes to identify sites which have been used before as 'virgin sites' are easier.
- Practise using the US on your colleagues – this will improve your anatomical knowledge.
- Be careful when suturing the line in position – this is where the most 'needlesticks' from this procedure occur!

should be contacted urgently. The wire needs to be removed as an emergency.

In the longer term any central line is a potential site for introduction of infection and for colonisation by micro-organisms.

Further reading

Hind D, Calvert N, McWilliams R, Davidson A, Paisley S, Beverley C, Thomas, S. (2003) Ultrasonic locating devices for central venous cannulation: meta-analysis. *Br Med J* 327: 361–70.

McGee DC, Gould MK. (2003) Current concepts: preventing complications of central venous catheterization. *N Engl J Med* 348: 1123–33.

National Institute for Health and Clinical Excellence. (2002) The clinical effectiveness and cost effectiveness of ultrasonic locating devices for the placement of central venous lines. *NICE technology appraisal guidance 49.* www.nice.org.uk/TA2

CHAPTER 12

Access: Emergency – Intraosseous Access and Venous Cutdown

Matt Boylan

Midlands Air Ambulance, DCAE Cosford, UK

OVERVIEW

By the end of this chapter you should be able to:

- understand the indications for intraosseous access and venous cutdown
- identify the sites used for intraosseous access and venous cutdown
- be aware of different types of intraosseous access devices
- describe the procedure of performing intraosseous access and venous cutdown
- understand the contraindications for intraosseous access and venous cutdown.

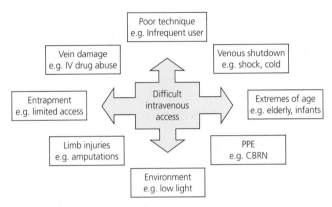
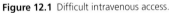

Figure 12.1 Difficult intravenous access.

Introduction

Gaining access to the circulatory system in the critically ill or injured patient is an essential part of the resuscitative process. Failure to do so can result in significant delays in the delivery of life-saving treatment. There are situations where peripheral intravenous access may be difficult or even impossible (Figure 12.1). Intraosseous access and venous cutdown are useful alternatives in this situation.

Where possible a full explanation of the proceedure should be given to the patient and informed consent gained. However, in many cases this will not be possible.

Intraosseous access

The intraosseous (IO) space consists of spongy cancellous epiphyseal bone and the diaphyseal medullary cavity. It houses a vast non-collapsible venous plexus that communicates with the arteries and veins of the systemic circulation via small channels in the surrounding compact cortical bone (Figure 12.2). Drugs or fluids administered into the intraosseous space via a needle or catheter will pass rapidly into the systemic circulation at a rate comparable with central or peripheral venous access. Any drug, fluid or blood product that can be given intravenously can be given via the intraosseous route.

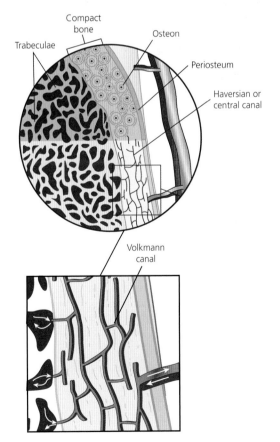

Figure 12.2 Osseous blood supply.

ABC of Practical Procedures. Edited by T. Nutbeam and R. Daniels. © 2010
Blackwell Publishing, ISBN: 978-1-4051-8595-0.

A marrow sample aspirated immediately following needle insertion can be used for biochemical (acid–base status, glucose, electrolytes) and/or haematological (haemoglobin, cross-match) testing. Test accuracy reduces following continuous infusion, drug administration and prolonged cardiac arrest.

Insertion pain due to stimulation of nociceptors in the skin and periosteum is equivalent to that of wide-bore peripheral intravenous access. Pain on initial infusion is due to intraosseous vessel wall distension and may be severe. It can be reduced in the conscious patient by the administration of 20–40 mg lidocaine (0.5 mg/kg paediatric) through the device before commencing an infusion.

Insertion site selection

The factors affecting IO insertion site selection include the type of device being used, the age/size of the patient, the presence or absence of contraindications to insertion (Box 12.1), and the skill of the operator.

Insertion sites

See Figure 12.3.

Sternum (manubrium)

One fingerbreadth (1.5 cm) below sternal notch in midline (adult). Sternal devices only.

Humerus (greater tubercle)

Adduct patient's arm, flex elbow and place their hand onto their umbilicus.

1 Palpate the anterior midshaft humerus. Continue palpating proximally up the anterior surface of the humerus until the greater tubercle is met.
2 Palpate coracoid and acromion. Imagine a line between them and drop a line approx 2 cm from its midpoint to the insertion site (adult/older child).

Pelvis (iliac crest)

Palpate the anterior superior iliac spine (ASIS); continue posterolaterally along iliac crest to the insertion point 5–6 cm from the ASIS (adult).

Distal femur (anterolateral surface)

3 cm above lateral femoral condyle (child).

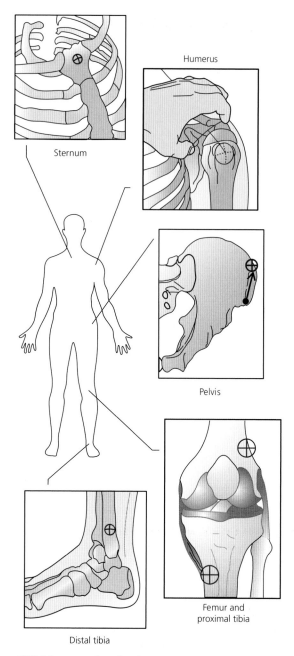

Figure 12.3 Intraosseous insertion sites.

Proximal tibia (anteromedial surface)

Adult: two fingerbreadths below and medial to the tibial tuberosity.

Child: one fingerbreadth below tibial tuberosity (or two fingerbreadths below patella) and then medial on flat aspect of tibia.

Distal tibia (medial surface)

Adult: two fingerbreadths proximal to the tip of the medial malleolus.

Child: one fingerbreadth proximal to the tip of the medial malleolus.

Box 12.2 **Complications of insertion of IO needle**

- Extravasation
- Compartment syndrome
- Osteomyelitis (0.6%)
- Fracture
- Fat embolism (rare)
- Growth plate injury (theoretical)

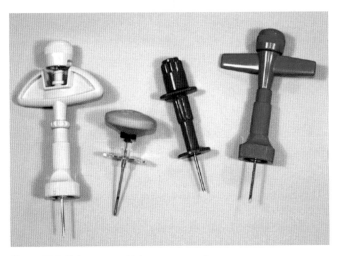

Figure 12.4 Various manual intraosseous needles.

NOTE—The recommended insertion site may differ between devices; therefore the manufacturer's guidelines should be consulted before use.

Complications of insertion (Box 12.2)

Extravasation of fluid may occur following incorrect insertion or needle dislodgment. If unrecognised, continued fluid leak into a limb compartment could result in compartment syndrome. There is a small risk of osteomyelitis (0.6%) and local cellulitis following intraosseous needle insertion. Most reported cases were associated with prolonged needle usage. It is therefore recommended that all IO needles should be removed within 24 hours of insertion. Fracture of the bone during needle insertion is rare unless the patient has brittle bones (osteoporosis/osteogenesis imperfecta). In these cases alternative methods of securing circulatory access should be considered. There is a theoretical risk of growth plate injury from insertion in children. Careful insertion site identification and angling the needle away from the growth plate following cortical penetration will reduce this risk.

Manual intraosseous needles

There are different variants of manual intraosseous needle (Figure 12.4). Until recently these were designed primarily for paediatric use. Their use in adults often failed due to bending or slipping of the needle on the harder adult cortex. More robust manual models are now available for use in adults (Figure 12.5). They are all hand-driven modified steel needles with removable stylets that prevent plugging with bone fragments during insertion. They

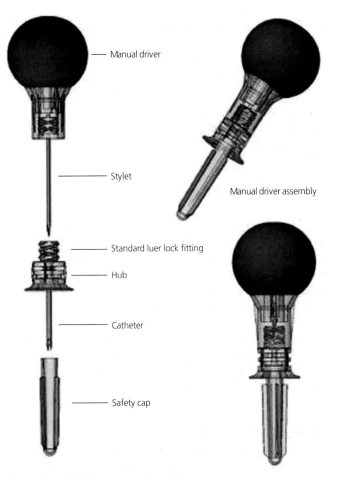

Figure 12.5 EZ-IO™ manual needle (adult).

have specially designed handles that allow the operator to push and rotate the needle through the hard cortical bone.

Step-by-step guide: manual intraosseous needles
(Figure 12.6)

1 Identify and clean insertion site.
2 Cup the handle in the palm of the hand and stabilise the needle with fingers.
3 Hold the device perpendicular to the bone surface.
4 Insert the needle through the skin and into the bone by rotating the needle set clockwise–counterclockwise and applying downward pressure.
5 Stop when you feel a pop/give. The needle tip should now lie in the intraosseous space.
6 Remove the stylet.
7 Attempt aspiration of a marrow sample.
8 Attach connector and flush system.
9 Support/protect needle in position.

Any rocking motion during insertion will enlarge the insertion hole and could lead to extravasation. A rapid flush following insertion will improve subsequent infusion rates through the device. Whilst there will be some flow due to gravity, the best infusion rates will be achieved using either a pressure infusion or by syringing. The latter is achieved by attaching a three-way tap and syringe into

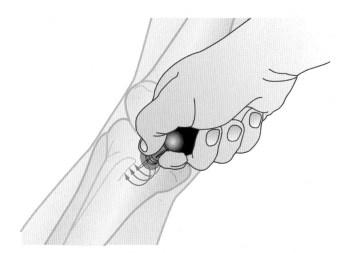

Figure 12.6 Manual needle insertion.

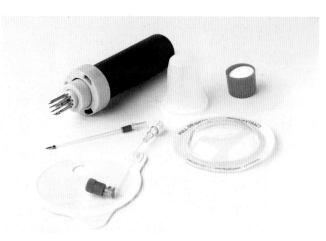

Figure 12.8 FAST1™ intraosseous infusion system.

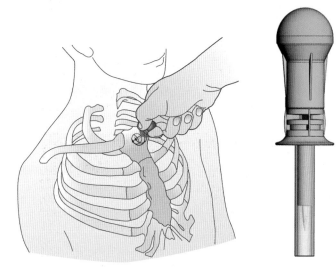

Figure 12.7 EZ-IO™ manual sternal needle.

the infusion line. Syringing also allows accurate fluid titration in children.

Manual sternal needle

A manual adult sternal intraosseous set (EZ-IO™ Sternal Intraosseous Set) is currently being trialled by the UK military. The device has a collar to limit the depth of needle penetration through the sternum. It requires a small skin incision for insertion in order to accommodate the collar. An adhesive needle stabiliser aids stability following insertion. Estimated insertion time is 30 seconds. See Figure 12.7.

Impact-driven intraosseous needles
FAST1™ intraosseous infusion system

The FAST1™ (Pyng Medical) is a disposable hand-held device that uses an internal spring mechanism to access the sternal medullary space (Figure 12.8). It can only be used on the adult sternum and utilises a target patch to indicate the insertion point on the manubrium. As pressure is applied to the device a central penetrating needle is fired precisely into the sternal medullary space. The

multiple needle design prevents the operator from accidentally penetrating through the sternum. Estimated time for insertion is 50 seconds.

Step-by-step guide: FAST-1 device
1 Locate and swab insertion site.
2 Align target patch with sternal notch (Figure 12.9a).
3 Holding device perpendicular to the surface of the manubrium place introducer needle cluster into target area (Figure 12.9b,c).
4 Increase pressure on device until the device releases.
5 Lift introducer device off inserted infusion tube.
6 Attach extension set and flush before use (Figure 12.9d).
7 Attach protective dome (Figure 12.9e).
  The sternal infusion tube should be removed within 24 hours. Insertion failures are mostly due to improper insertion technique (i.e. not inserting perpendicular to manubrium) or patient obesity.

Bone injection gun (BIG™)
The BIG™ is a light-weight, self-contained device that comes in both adult and paediatric models (Figure 12.10). It is licensed for use on the distal and proximal tibia and the humerus. When correctly triggered a powerful spring fires the needle a preset distance into the medullary space. The appropriate insertion depth is selected by the operator. Estimated time for insertion is 17 seconds.

Step-by-step guide: bone injection gun (Figure 12.11)
1 Set correct insertion depth.
2 Locate and clean insertion site.
3 Hold the barrel of the device (arrowed) firmly against insertion point at 90° to the bone surface.
4 Squeeze and pull out red safety latch.
5 Apply pressure with the free hand to top of device to fire the needle.
6 Slowly remove the device from the inserted needle.
7 Remove the needle trocar.
8 Attach extension set and flush before use.
9 Support and protect insertion site.

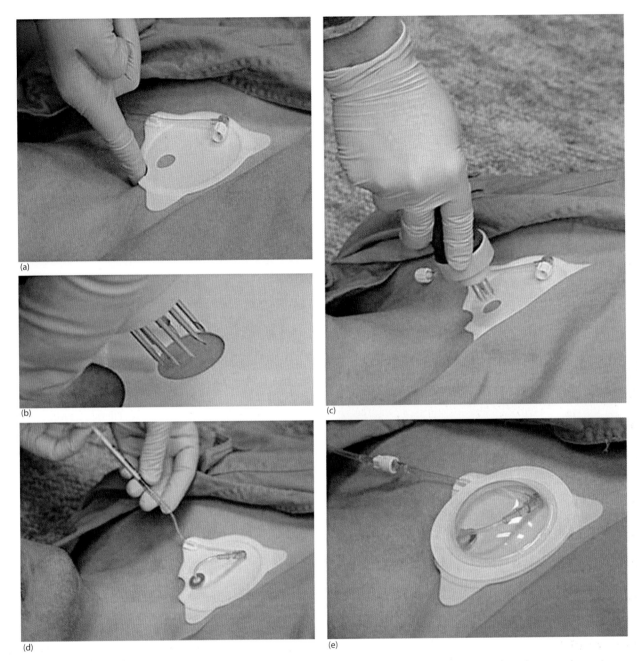

(a)

(b)

(c)

(d)

(e)

Figure 12.9 FAST1™ insertion.

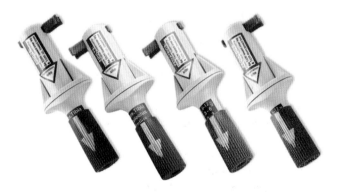

Figure 12.10 BIG™ – adult and paediatric.

The needle should be removed within 24 hours by careful twisting using forceps. The preset insertion site and depth markings may be inadequate for some patients, leading to failure of the needle to penetrate the medullary cavity. The device should be placed against the insertion site before the safety latch is removed to reduce the risk of accidental firing.

Drill-driven intraosseous needles
EZ-IO™ intraosseous infusion system

The EZ-IO intraosseous infusion system uses a hand-held power drill to drive a hollow drill-tipped needle into the intraosseous space (Figure 12.12). The EZ-IO™ needles come in both adult AD (25-mm; 15G) and Paediatric PD (15-mm 15G) sizes (Figure 12.13).

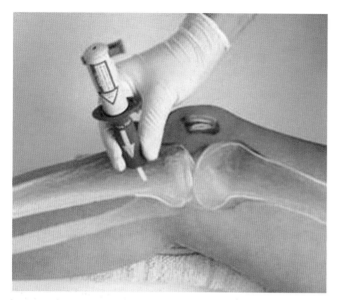

Figure 12.11 BIG™ insertion.

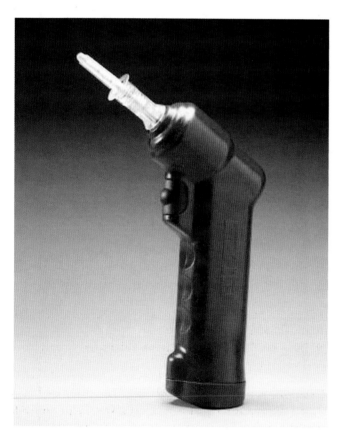

Figure 12.12 EZ-IO™ power driver.

The stainless steel drill-tipped needles have a more precise and tight fit once inserted than needles inserted manually or by impact-driven devices. This reduces the incidence of extravasation. The device is licensed for use on the proximal and distal tibia and humeral head. It has also been used in the iliac crest. Estimated insertion time is 10 seconds.

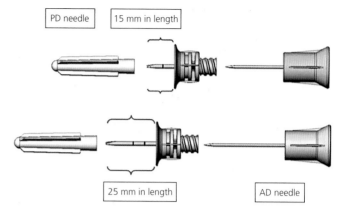

Figure 12.13 EZ-IO™ needles.

Step-by-step guide: drill-driven intraosseous needles

1 Identify and clean insertion site (Figure 12.14a,b).
2 Attach appropriate needle to driver (magnetic).
3 Remove needle safety cap.
4 Stabilise insertion site.
5 Insert needle perpendicular to bone.
6 Drill until hit bone – check 5 mm mark (Figure 12.14c).
7 Continue drilling until you feel a give/pop.
8 Remove the driver from the needle.
9 Unscrew the stylet from the needle (Figure 12.14d).
10 Attach the extension set.
11 Aspirate then flush (Figure 12.14e).

Each needle has a black line 5 mm from the flange. This should be visible at or above skin level after the needle has been driven through the skin and is touching the bone. If the mark is not visible then the needle set may not be long enough to reach the intraosseous space and an alternative site should be selected. The needle should be removed within 24 hours by attaching a Luer-Lok™ syringe to the needle hub and twisting clockwise whilst applying traction (Figure 12.14f).

Summary

Intraosseous access is an accepted means of gaining emergency access to the circulatory system in the paediatric patient. The development of stronger needles and mechanical insertion devices has allowed for its use in adults too. It is quicker, safer and requires less skill to perform than central venous cannulation. It should be the method of choice for emergency access when peripheral cannulation is difficult or has failed.

Venous cutdown

Venous cutdown is a surgical technique by which a selected vein is exposed and mobilised and then cannulated under direct vision. It has been largely replaced by central venous and intraosseous access, but remains a useful alternative when other methods fail or are not available.

Cutdown sites (Figure 12.15)
Basilic vein (antecubital fossa)
Adult: 2–3 cm lateral to the medial epicondyle of the humerus.

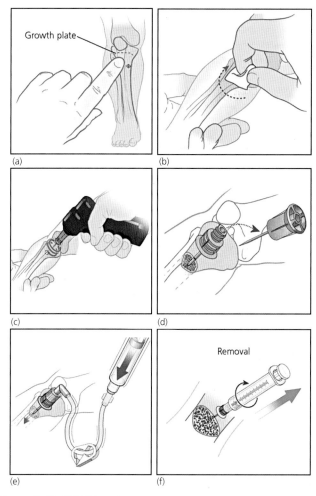

Figure 12.14 EZ-IO™ insertion.

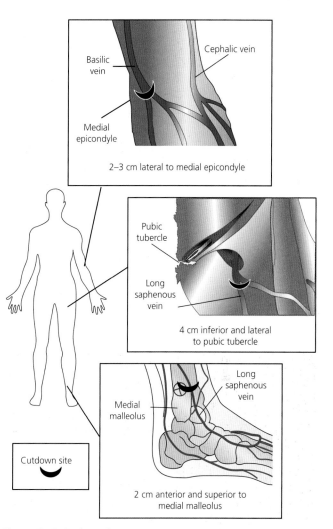

Figure 12.15 Cutdown sites.

Child: 1–2 cm lateral to the medial epicondyle of the humerus.

Long saphenous vein (groin)
Adult: 4 cm inferior and lateral to the pubic tubercle.

Long saphenous vein (ankle)
Adult: 2 cm anterior and superior to the medial malleolus.
Child: 1 cm anterior and superior to the medial malleolus.

Step-by-step guide: cutdown method (Figure 12.16)
1 Place a venous tourniquet proximal to intended cutdown site where possible.
2 Identify cutdown site and inject local anaesthetic along the intended incision line if the patient is conscious.
3 Make a transverse incision through skin being careful not to damage the underlying vein (Figure 12.16a).
4 Spread the skin and identify the vein lying at right angles to the line of the incision. Mobilise a 2-cm length of vein by blunt dissection using curved forceps (Figure 12.16b).
5 Pull a loop of suture (e.g. 2/0 vicryl) under vein (Figure 12.16c). Cut the loop to form proximal and distal sutures.

6 Tie off distal suture and transfix vein with a needle (Figure 12.16d).
7 Make a vertical stab incision down onto the transfixing needle to produce a hole (venotomy) in the anterior vein wall (Figure 12.16e).
8 Insert a cannula or the cut end of a sterile giving set through venotomy into vein (Figure 12.16f).
9 Tie off proximal suture around vein and inserted cannula.
10 Suture and dress wound.

Complications
The risk of complications with venous cutdown is higher than with peripheral cannulation and intraosseous access (Box 12.3).

Access to the vein may prove difficult in obese patients due to increased amount of adipose tissue. Incisions may need to be extended in order to gain adequate exposure.

Damage to adjacent nerves and vessels can occur during the procedure. The saphenous nerve is often damaged during cutdown attempts at the ankle.

Even with good exposure cannulation of the vein can be difficult. It is easy to perforate the posterior vein wall when making a venotomy in a collapsed shutdown peripheral vein. Transfixing the

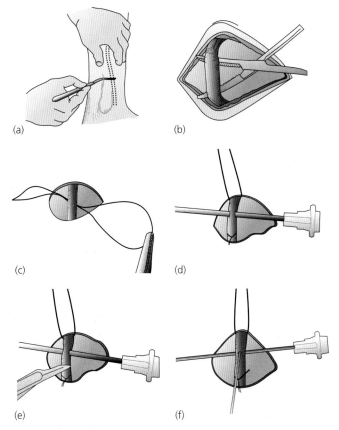

Figure 12.16 Cutdown method.

Handy hints/troubleshooting

- These skills are rarely used and therefore difficult to practise. The first time you perform this procedure may be for 'real'.
- Watch videos and practice on mannequins so you are familiar with the technique and equipment used.
- If you are appropriately trained, don't be afraid to use your skills in an emergency.

vein with a needle and cutting down onto the needle will prevent this in most cases.

Summary

Venous cutdown can be a useful technique when peripheral access fails and intraosseous access is unavailable. It does carry with it a greater morbidity, but this may be outweighed by the need for circulatory access in the unwell patient.

Further reading

Bone injection gun™ www.waismed.com

Chappell S, Vilke G, Chan T, Harrigan R, Ufberg J. (2006) Peripheral venous cutdown. *JEM* 31(4): 411–16.

EZ-IO™ intraosseous infusion system. www.vidacare.com

FAST1™ intraosseous infusion system. www.pyng.com

Lavis M, Vaghela A, Tozer C. (2000) Adult intraosseous infusion in accident and emergency departments in the UK. *EMJ* 17: 29–32.

McIntosh BB, Dulchavsky SA. Peripheral vascular cutdown. (1992) *Crit Care Clin* 8: 807–18.

CHAPTER 13

Therapeutic: Airway – Basic Airway Manoeuvres and Adjuncts

Tim Nutbeam

West Midlands School of Emergency Medicine, Birmingham, UK

OVERVIEW

By the end of this chapter you should be able to:
- identify a partially obstructed or blocked airway
- apply a head-tilt/chin-lift and jaw thrust
- describe how to size and insert oropharyngeal (OP) and nasopharyngeal (NP) airways
- describe how to ventilate a patient using a bag-valve-mask technique.

Introduction

Basic airway manoeuvres are life-saving. They are simple to do, easily learnt and should be readily performed by all healthcare practitioners. Airway adjuncts are available throughout nearly all clinical settings; familiarity with their use is vital. Many patients requiring these procedures are critically ill, and senior and/or specialist support should be sought at the earliest opportunity.

The obstructed or blocked airway

It is critical to identify an obstructed or blocked airway and provide immediate intervention. The airway should be assessed using a look, listen and feel approach.

Look for:
- evidence of obstruction in the airway: blood, vomit, foreign body, chewing gum, etc.
- adequate chest movement
- tracheal tug: indicating a completely obstructed airway.

Listen for:
- noisy breathing on inspiration (stridor) or expiration
- the absence of air movement.

Feel for:
- adequate chest movement
- air movement at the lips.

ABC of Practical Procedures. Edited by T. Nutbeam and R. Daniels. © 2010
Blackwell Publishing, ISBN: 978-1-4051-8595-0.

The airway is most commonly obstructed by the tongue in an unconscious patient – it falls backwards to obstruct the pharynx.

Airway manoeuvres

These manoeuvres are designed to displace the tongue anteriorly, bringing it forward out of the pharynx and clearing the airway.

Indications
- An obstructed or blocked airway.
- To assist in ventilation of an unconscious patient.
- Preparation for or to assist in advanced airway manoeuvres.

Contraindications
- Patients who have potential or actual cervical spine injury should not have a head-tilt/chin-lift as this may exacerbate their injuries: a jaw thrust should be applied as an alternative.

Head-tilt/chin-lift
1 Place the fingers of one hand under the mandible, gently lift the chin forward.
2 Use the thumb of the same hand to depress the lower lip and to open the mouth.

The position you are trying to achieve is the 'sniffing the morning air' position seen in Figure 13.1.

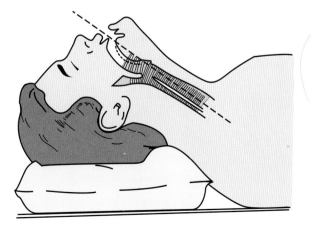

Figure 13.1 An open airway 'sniffing the morning air position'.

Jaw thrust

1 Place the fingers of both hands under the corresponding side of the mandible, at the angle of the jaw.
2 Lift the mandible forwards, opening the airway (avoid moving the patient's head).

Airway adjuncts

Use of airway adjuncts can assist in obtaining or maintaining an unobstructed, open airway.

Oropharyngeal airway

An oropharyngeal (OP) airway is designed to hold the tongue away from the posterior pharynx; this allows passage of air both through the device itself and around it (Figure 13.2).

An oropharyngeal airway consists of three parts: a flange, the body and the tip (Figure 13.3).

The flange protrudes from the patient's mouth. Its shape prevents the airway slipping further into the oropharynx.

The body is made from rigid plastic anatomically designed to fit the contour of the hard palate. It curves over the top of the patient's tongue.

The tip sits at the base of the tongue allowing air passage through and around the airway.

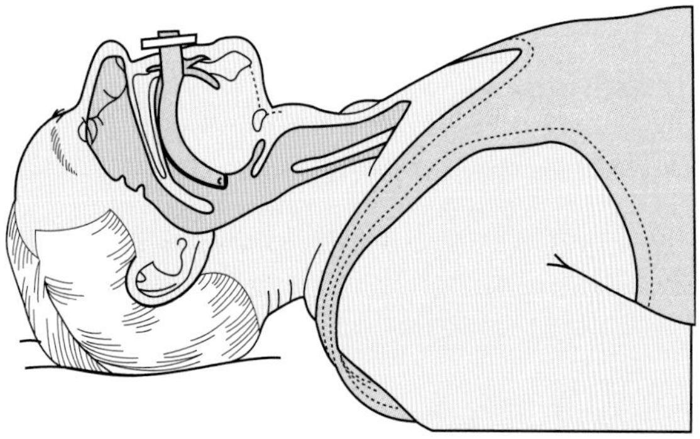

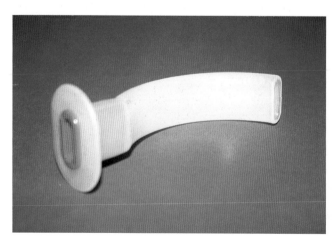

Figure 13.2 A correctly positioned OP airway.

Figure 13.3 OP airway showing flange, body and tip.

Indications

- Maintaining an airway opened by a head-tilt/chin-lift or jaw thrust.
- As an alternative method of opening an obstructed airway when airway manoeuvres have failed.
- As a 'bite-block' to protect an endotracheal tube.

Contraindications

- Patients must be unconscious to tolerate an OP airway. Inserting an airway in a semi-conscious patient may stimulate the gag reflex causing them to vomit, leading to further airway compromise and potential aspiration.

Sizing

- A correctly sized airway will extend from the corner of the patient's mouth to the angle of the mandible (Figure 13.4).
- Improper sizing can cause bleeding of the airway and obstruction of the glottis.

Step-by-step guide: oropharyngeal airway

1 Choose an appropriately sized airway (Figure 13.4).
2 Open the patient's mouth (if an assistant is available get them to do a jaw thrust).
3 Insert the airway upside down, with the curvature towards the tongue and the tip towards the hard palate (Figure 13.5a).
4 When the airway reaches the back of the tongue, rotate the device 180° so the tip faces downwards (Figure 13.5b).
5 Ensure the patient's tongue/lips are not caught between the airway and the teeth (Figure 13.5c).
6 Reassess the patient's airway for patency.

Nasopharyngeal (NP) airway

Similar to an OP airway, the nasopharyngeal (NP) airway is designed to hold the tongue away from the posterior pharynx (Figure 13.6).

The NP airway consists of the flange, the shaft and the bevel (Figure 13.7). All are made of soft flexible plastic to prevent trauma

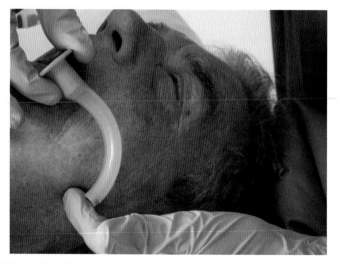

Figure 13.4 Sizing an OP airway. Measured from the incisors to the angle of the jaw.

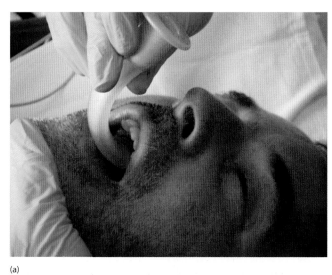

(a)

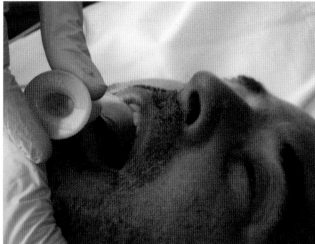

(b)

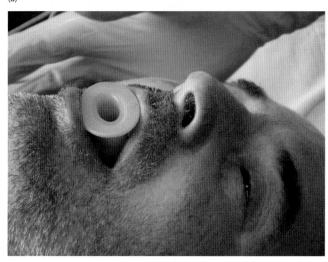

(c)

Figure 13.5 Step-by-step guide: OP airway. (a) Inserting the airway 'upside down'. (b) Rotation of airway. (c) Final position of airway.

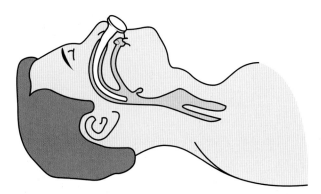

Figure 13.6 Position of a correctly inserted NP airway.

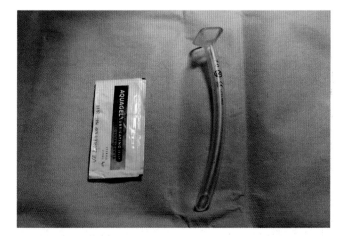

Figure 13.7 Equipment: NP airway and lubricant.

to the patient. Most NP airways require a safety pin inserted through the flange to prevent the airway slipping into the oropharynx.

Indications

- Maintaining an airway opened by a head-tilt/chin-lift or jaw thrust.
- As an alternative method of opening an obstructed airway when airway manoeuvres have failed.
- Better tolerated than OP airways in semi-conscious patients.
- Excellent for use in patients unable to open their mouths (e.g. trismus or seizures).
- As a means of facilitating bronchial suction.

Contraindications

- Known or potential base of skull fracture
- Commonly causes nose bleeds so should be avoided in those patients known to have bleeding tendencies (e.g. on warfarin).

Sizing

- NP airways were traditionally sized choosing a diameter which closest matched that of the patient's little finger (Figure 13.8). A better 'fit' is achieved using the chart in Table 13.1.

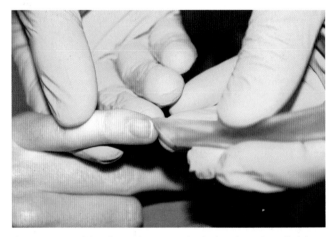

Figure 13.8 Traditionally NP airways are sized using the patient's little finger.

Table 13.1 Appropriate-sized NP airways.

Patient	Size of NP (diameter)
Average-height female	6
Average-height male	7
Large male	8

Step-by-step guide: nasopharyngeal airway

1 Choose an appropriately sized NP airway.
2 If necessary, place a safety pin through the flange of the NP (this ensures it does not fully enter the nasal cavity).
3 Apply a water-based lubricant (Figure 13.9a).
4 Insert the NP airway into the right nostril first (unless blocked, nasogastric tube in situ etc.) (Figure 13.9b). The bevel should be on the medial side of the NP airway.
5 The NP airway should be inserted at 90° to the patient's forehead, and should pass with minimal resistance towards the patient's occiput.
6 Rolling the NP from side to side in your fingers as you exert downwards pressure may make insertion easier (Figure 13.9c,d).
7 If resistance is met try the other nostril.
8 Reassess the patient's airway for patency.

Bag-valve-mask (with reservoir)

In many patients a simple airway manoeuvre or use of an adjunct to open the airway will allow them to breathe spontaneously. If this is the case high-flow oxygen (15L/min) should be administered via a mask with non-rebreathe reservoir.

If they are not breathing sufficiently it is necessary to ventilate the patient. The most convenient method of achieving this is with a bag-valve-mask with reservoir. This device consists of the following.

- *A tight fitting face mask.* This facemask must be appropriately sized to the patient and allow an airtight seal between the mask and the patient's face.
- *A self-filling chamber.* Usually 2 litres in size, this chamber is self-filling. The chamber will preferentially fill from the oxygen reservoir, but in the absence of an oxygen supply still allows the patient to be ventilated on room air (21% O_2).
- *A one-way valve.* This allows oxygen (or air) to be entrained into the self-filling chamber and then applied as a positive pressure to ventilate the patient.
- *An oxygen reservoir.* This oxygen reservoir fills when the valve is closed and is used to fill the bag when the valve is open.
- *Tubing.* To connect the reservoir and chamber to an oxygen supply.

Step-by-step guide: bag-valve-mask

1 Assemble the bag-valve-mask with an appropriately sized face mask for the patient.
2 Connect the tubing to a high-flow oxygen supply (15L).
3 Ensure the reservoir fully inflates with oxygen.
4 Check the valve is closed and opens when the chamber is squeezed.
5 Place the face mask on the patient ensuring a tight seal (do not remove any airway adjuncts).
6 Apply a head-tilt/chin-lift or jaw thrust to the patient.
7 Squeeze the chamber at a rate of 10–12 breaths a minute.
8 Ensure adequate ventilation by bilateral chest movement and fogging of the face mask on expiration.

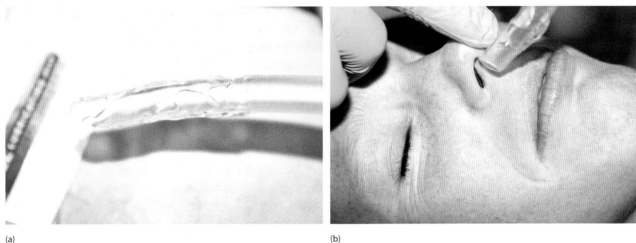

(a)

(b)

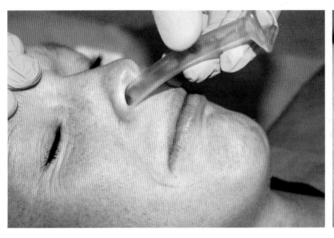

(c)

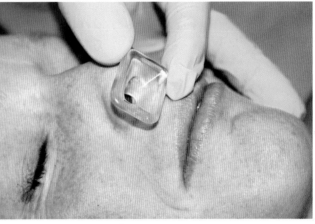

(d)

Figure 13.9 Step-by-step guide: NP airway. (a) Lubrication of NP airway. (b) Insertion of airway. (c) Partial insertion: roll between fingers. (d) NP airway in position.

Handy hints/troubleshooting

- A supervised session with an experienced anaesthetist is an ideal environment to learn and practice these life-saving procedures.
- If you have difficulty ventilating a patient use two hands to hold the mask/perform the jaw thrust and get an assistant to squeeze the chamber of the bag-valve-mask.
- Ensure the oxygen reservoir is fully inflated on the bag-valve-mask and connected to the oxygen supply (*not AIR!*).
- NP airways tend to be better tolerated than OP airways in patients with fluctuating consciousness.

Further reading

American College of Surgeons. (2008) Advanced Trauma Life Support: Student Manual, 8th edn.

Dolenska S, Dalal P, Taylor A. (2004) *Essentials of airway management.* Greenwich Medical Media, London.

Resuscitation Council UK. (2006) Airway management and ventilation. In: *Advanced Life Support Course-Provider Manual, 5th edn.* Resuscitation Council UK, London.

CHAPTER 14

Therapeutic: Airway – Insertion of Laryngeal Mask Airway

Tim Nutbeam

West Midlands School of Emergency Medicine, Birmingham, UK

> **OVERVIEW**
>
> By the end of this chapter you should be able to:
> - understand the indications for inserting a laryngeal mask airway (LMA®)
> - be aware of the various types of LMA
> - describe how to size and insert a LMA
> - understand the benefits and limitations of the LMA.

Introduction

The laryngeal mask airway has an important role in advanced airway management. It is recommended for use in patients requiring advanced life support and is relatively easily inserted by the non-specialist.

Indications

- A first-line airway management device in those with limited airway management experience.
- Airway management in an unconscious patient who requires assisted ventilation in the absence of the ability to provide a definitive airway.
- As an alternative to oropharyngeal and nasopharyngeal airways (more suitable for prolonged ventilation).
- Emergency airway management at a cardiorespiratory arrest.
- Suitable airway device for certain operations/anaesthetics.
- Part of a 'failed intubation' drill (alternative to ET tube).

Contraindications

- When a definitive airway (cuffed tube in the trachea) is required.
- High-risk anaesthetics.
- Patient with fluctuating consciousness level (intact gag reflex is a contraindication due to risk of inducing vomiting).
- Unconscious patients unable to open mouth (e.g. trismus).
- Patients requiring high airway pressure to ventilate (e.g. heavily pregnant, obese, asthmatic).

ABC of Practical Procedures. Edited by T. Nutbeam and R. Daniels. © 2010
Blackwell Publishing, ISBN: 978-1-4051-8595-0.

Anatomy

The anatomy of the pharynx and larynx has been covered in Chapter 15. The LMA when inserted correctly sits at the interface between the trachea and the oesophagus. Here it forms a low-pressure seal around the glottis (see Figure 14.1).

Equipment

The LMA exists in a multitude of forms. The basic LMA consists of the following (Figure 14.2).

- *15-mm connector.* This is a standard connector which will attach to a bag-valve-mask, ventilator, filter etc.
- *Tube.* An anatomically designed semi-flexible tube. A black line often runs along the back of the airway enabling easy orientation (should face towards the practitioner at the 'head' end).
- *Inflation port.* The volume of air to be injected through this one-way valve can be found in Table 14.1. It is important to note that LMAs are removed fully inflated (unlike an ET tube where the cuff is fully deflated before removal).
- *Aperture bars.* These prevent the airway becoming obstructed by the patient's epiglottis (not universal).
- *Cuff.* An inflatable cuff, anatomically designed to form a low-pressure seal with minimal mucosal pressure.

Variations upon the 'classic' LMA exist which have been designed with additional features:

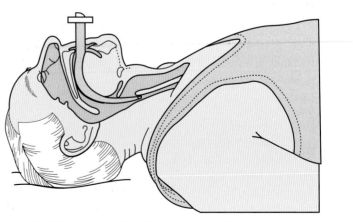

Figure 14.1 The position of the LMA when correctly inserted.

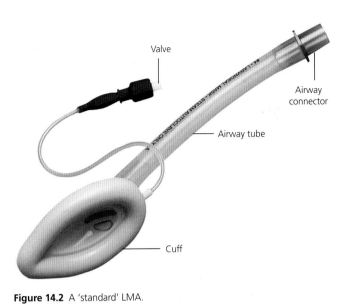

Figure 14.2 A 'standard' LMA.

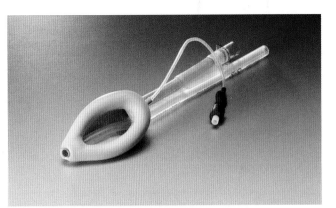

Figure 14.4 Pro-seal LMA.

Table 14.1

LMA size	Type	Weight	Inflation volume
3	Small adult	30–50 kg	20 mL
4	Normal adult	50–70 kg	30 mL
5	Large adult	70 kg+	40 mL

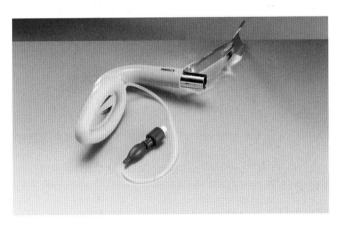

Figure 14.3 Intubating LMA.

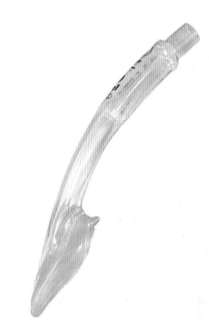

Figure 14.5 I-gel Supraglottic Device.

Sizing

A guide to choosing the correct size of LMA can be found in Table 14.1.

Step-by-step guide: laryngeal mask airway

1 Preoxygenate the patient using the bag-valve-mask technique described in Chapter 13 (Figure 14.6a).
2 Deflate or partly deflate the cuff of the LMA and apply a water-soluble lubricant to the posterior surface of the cuff.
3 Hold the LMA like a pencil in your dominant hand, with the index finger placed at the junction of the cuff and the tube.
4 Place your non-dominant hand on the back of the patient's head. Extend the head (unless cervical spine instability is suspected or known) and flex the neck (Figure 14.6b).
5 Press the tip of the cuff up against the hard palate and flatten the cuff against it (it helps to rotate the cuff slightly laterally at this point).
6 Use your index finger to guide the cuff down towards your non-dominant hand (Figure 14.6c).

Intubating LMA (iLMA®)—A modification of the original LMA through which an endotracheal tube can be passed blindly (Figure 14.3). For use in difficult airways.

Pro-seal LMA®—A drain tube provides direct access to drain stomach contents; this reduces the incidence of aspiration (Figure 14.4).

I-gel® Supraglottic Airway—This variant does not have a cuff that requires inflation. It also incorporates a gastric channel and an integral bite block to reduce the possibility of airway occlusion (Figure 14.5).

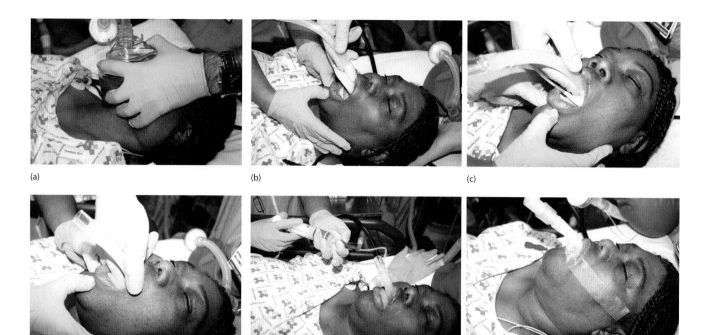

Figure 14.6 Step-by-step guide: laryngeal mask airway. (a) Preoxygenating the patient with high-concentration oxygen. (b) Insertion of LMA whilst a trained assistant provides a jawthrust. (c) Insertion of LMA with correct finger position. (d) Advancement of LMA until resistance is felt. (e) Inflation of cuff. (f) LMA secured in position with tape.

7 Advance the LMA into the hypopharynx until a definite resistance is felt (Figure 14.6d).
8 Inflate the cuff with just enough air to obtain a seal. As the cuff inflates it tends to 'pop up' slightly into the correct position (Figure 14.6e).
9 Connect the LMA to your means of ventilation.
10 Confirm adequate ventilation using the 'look, listen, feel' approach described in the previous chapter.
11 Secure the LMA with tape or ribbon.

Handy hints/troubleshooting

• A supervised session with an experienced anaesthetist is an ideal environment to learn and practice this procedure.
• A size 4 LMA is suitable for most females and a size 5 for most males.
• Deflate the cuff fully before use (they are sometimes provided partially inflated).
• If the patient does not tolerate the LMA remove it with the cuff fully inflated.

Further reading

Dolenska S, Dalal P, Taylor A. (2004) *Essentials of Airway Management.* Greenwich Medical Media, London.
Resuscitation Council UK. (2006) Airway management and ventilation. In: *Advanced Life Support Course-Provider Manual*, 5th edn. Resuscitation Council UK, London.

CHAPTER 15

Therapeutic: Endotracheal Intubation

Randeep Mullhi

Department of Anaesthesia, Queen Elizabeth Hospital, Birmingham, UK

OVERVIEW

By the end of this chapter you should understand:

- indications for tracheal intubation and associated complications
- anatomy of pharynx, larynx and trachea
- how to perform tracheal intubation
- the difficult airway and strategies for management
- the surgical airway
- situations requiring the use of cricoid pressure.

Introduction

Tracheal intubation is considered the optimal method of securing a patient's airway. It involves placing a cuffed tube in the trachea.

Indications

- Protection from aspiration, e.g. in patients with decreased Glasgow Coma Score (<8) due to head injury or anaesthesia.
- Where positive pressure ventilation is required, e.g. in patients undergoing neurosurgery following intracranial bleed.
- Cardiorespiratory arrest.
- Restricted access to the patient, e.g. maxofacial surgery, helicopter transport etc.

Anatomy of pharynx, larynx and trachea

The pharynx is the common upper end of the respiratory and gastrointestinal tracts. It is a fibromuscular tube extending from the base of the skull to the level of the C6 vertebra. It then continues as the oesophagus.

The pharynx is divided into:

- *nasopharynx*, which lies behind the nasal cavity but above the soft palate
- *oropharynx*, which lies behind the mouth and tongue and extends from the soft palate to the tip of the epiglottis

- *laryngopharynx*, which lies behind and around the larynx. It extends from the level of the epiglottic tip to the C6 level where it becomes continuous with the oesophagus. The larynx projects into the laryngopharynx forming a deep recess (the pyriform fossa) on each side (Figure 15.1).

The larynx lies between the pharynx and trachea, extending from C3 to the C6 vertebra. It is composed of hyoid bone and epiglottic, thyroid, cricoid, arytenoid, cuneiform and corniculate cartilages. These are joined by numerous muscles and ligaments (Figure 15.2).

The trachea is a continuation of the larynx. It is approximately 10 cm long and 2 cm wide in the adult. It is attached by the cricotracheal ligament to the lower level of the cricoid cartilage at the level of the C6 vertebra. It continues downwards to bifurcate into left and right main bronchi at the level of T4 (Figure 15.3).

Equipment

Laryngoscope

A laryngoscope consists of a handle and blade. A curved Macintosh blade is most often used. The most frequently used design has a bulb screwed on to the blade. The battery is housed in the handle. An electrical connection is made when the blade is opened ready for use (Figure 15.4).

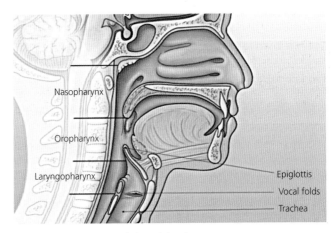

Figure 15.1 Cross-sectional view of the pharynx.

ABC of Practical Procedures. Edited by T. Nutbeam and R. Daniels. © 2010
Blackwell Publishing, ISBN: 978-1-4051-8595-0.

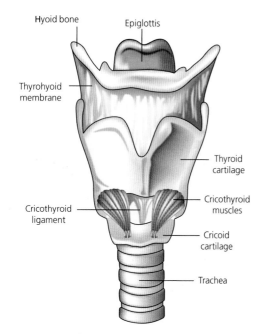

Figure 15.2 Structure of the larynx.

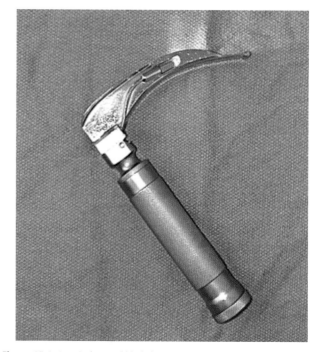

Figure 15.4 A typical curved blade laryngoscope.

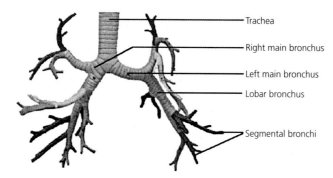

Figure 15.3 Trachea and its bifurcation into left and right main bronchi: the right main bronchus is wider and more vertical than the left. It is therefore more prone to being intubated if an endotracheal tube is advanced too far.

Cuffed tracheal tubes

Tubes used for intubation are single use and usually made of PVC. The internal diameter is marked on the outside of the tube in millimetres.

The tube is cut down to size to suit the individual patient, the length being marked on the outside in centimetres.

Cuffed tracheal tubes are used in adults. When inflated, the cuff forms a tight seal between the tube and tracheal wall. It protects the patient's airway against aspiration. The cuff is connected to a pilot balloon at the proximal end of the tube. After intubation the cuff is inflated via the pilot balloon until no gas leak can be heard during ventilation (Figure 15.5).

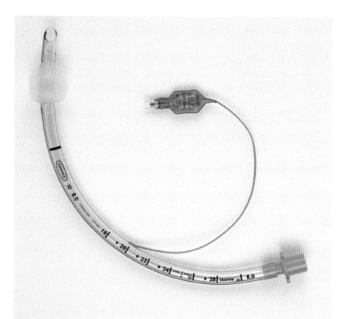

Figure 15.5 A typical PVC endotracheal tube. Current advanced life support guidelines recommend the use of a size 8.0 mm internal diameter tube in an adult male and a size 7.0 mm tube in an adult female. However, a range of tube sizes should be available appropriate to the size of the patient.

Additional equipment

In addition to the equipment mentioned above, adjuncts to intubation especially with difficult or potentially difficult airways are commonly used. This equipment includes the gum elastic

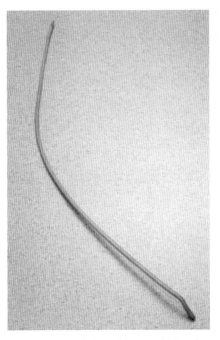

Figure 15.6 Gum elastic bougie: this device is used when the vocal cords are difficult to visualise completely. It is inserted through the cords and then the tracheal tube railroaded over it.

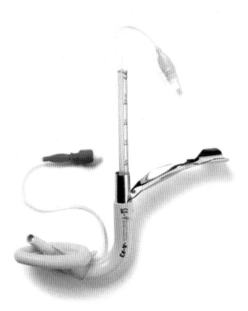

Figure 15.8 Intubating laryngeal mask airway (LMA): a modification of the original LMA through which an endotracheal tube can be passed blindly. The position of the mask cuff above the glottis when placed correctly acts as a conduit to the vocal cords.

> **Box 15.1 Equipment required for intubation**
>
> - Laryngoscope with selection of blades and spare batteries.
> - A selection of ET tubes.
> - Water-soluble jelly to lubricate the cuff to aid passage through the cords.
> - Tape to secure the tube in position.
> - A stethoscope to confirm the correct placement of the tube.
> - Suction apparatus should be available in case of regurgitation.
> - Intubation aids: gum elastic bougie and stylet.
> - Magills forceps.
> - A selection of oropharyngeal airways and laryngeal mask airways.
> - A means of detecting expired CO_2 should be used to confirm correct tube placement.

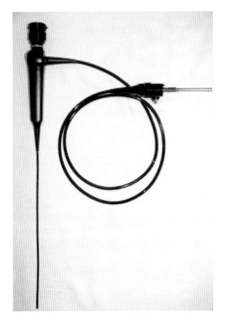

Figure 15.7 Fibreoptic laryngoscope: this device is used to visualise the patient's airway. A tracheal tube can be railroaded on to the scope and advanced off it once the vocal cords have been passed.

bougie (Figure 15.6), the fibreoptic laryngoscope (Figure 15.7) and the intubation laryngeal mask airway (iLMA) (Figure 15.8).

Step-by-step guide: orotracheal intubation

Prepare your equipment as per Box 15.1.

1 Preoxygenate the patient: intubation should be preceded by ventilation with the highest oxygen concentration possible. The intubation attempt should only take 30 seconds before re-oxygenating the patient.

2 Position: the neck is flexed slightly and the head extended to produce the classic 'sniffing the morning air position.' A pillow is placed under the head (Figure 15.9).

3 Insert the laryngoscope: the laryngoscope is held in the left hand. Introduce it gently at the right side of the mouth over the tongue. Important landmarks must be identified when advancing the laryngoscope into its correct position in the vallecula (see Box 15.2 & Figures 15.10, 15.11a).

4 With the blade of the laryngoscope in the vallecula, lift upwards along the line of the laryngoscope handle, avoiding pivoting on the upper teeth (Figure 15.11b). This lifts the epiglottis and should reveal the vocal cords. These are whitish in colour with their apex anteriorly (Figure 15.12).

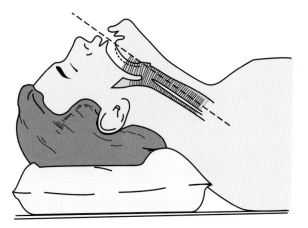

Figure 15.9 The 'sniffing the morning air' position in which the neck is slightly flexed with the head extended. This allows a direct line of vision from mouth to vocal cords.

Box 15.2 **Anatomical landmarks as you advance laryngoscope**

The tonsillar fossa: with the laryngoscope over the right side of the tongue, advance until the end of the soft palate appears to meet the lateral pharyngeal wall at the tonsillar fossa.

Uvula: push the tongue into the midline by moving the blade to the left. Using the posterior edge of the soft palate as a guide, advance the scope until the uvula is identified in the midline.

Epiglottis: advance the laryngoscope further over the base of the tongue until the tip of the epiglottis comes into view.

The laryngoscope should end up sitting in the vallecula. This is the area between the root of the epiglottis and the base of the tongue.

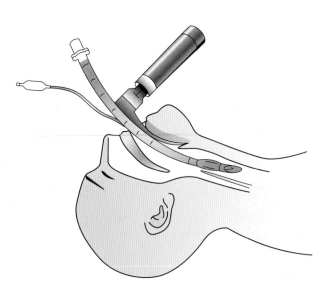

Figure 15.10 Correct position of the laryngoscope when sited in the vallecula.

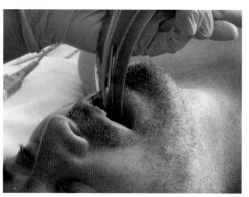

(a)

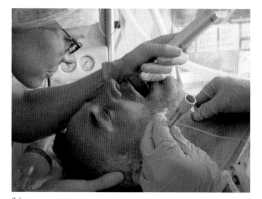

(b)

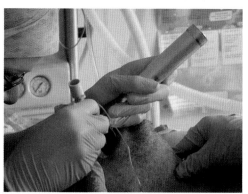

(c)

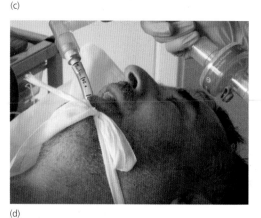

(d)

Figure 15.11 Step-by-step guide: orotracheal intubation. (a) Insertion of the laryngoscope making sure to avoid causing damage to the teeth. (b) Laryngoscopy with cricoid pressure. (c) Inserting the endotracheal tube. (d) The endotracheal tube secured with a tie.

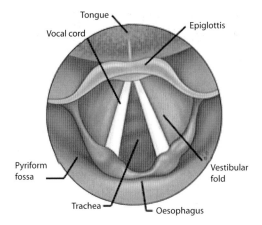

Figure 15.12 View of vocal cords at laryngoscopy.

Box 15.3 **Endotracheal tube position confirmation**

- Correct tube position is confirmed with the **look, listen and feel** approach. An end-tidal CO_2 monitor will confirm the presence in the trachea.
- **Look** for adequate chest movement.
- **Listen** for breath sounds over the precordium.
- **Feel** for chest expansion.

Remember: if in any doubt take the tube out!

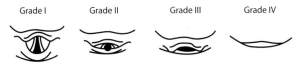

Figure 15.13 Cormack and Lehane classification of view at laryngoscopy. Grade I full view of vocal cords. Grade II partial view of vocal cords. Grade III only epiglottis seen. Grade IV epiglottis not seen. Grades III and IV are termed difficult.

5 Introduce the tube through the right side of the mouth. It is helpful to have an assistant pull on the right-hand corner of the mouth to give an improved view.

6 Advance the tube keeping the larynx in view until the cuff is positioned below the cords (Figure 15.11c). It is usually advanced to a depth of 23 cm at the incisors in an adult male and 21 cm in an adult female.

7 The tube is then connected to a means of ventilation such as a bag-valve-mask, a portable ventilator or an anaesthetic machine.

8 Inflate the cuff; the cuff should be inflated using a 20-mL syringe with room air. The cuff should be inflated until no leak around the cuff occurs with positive pressure ventilation.

9 Confirm the position of the tube, using a look, listen and feel approach (Box 15.3).

10 Secure the endotracheal tube using a tie or bandage (Figure 15.11d).

Difficulty with intubation

This can be predicted or completely unanticipated. A widely accepted classification of difficulty of intubation is related to the

Box 15.4 **Causes of difficult intubation**

- Inexperienced practitioner.
- Difficulty inserting the laryngoscope (e.g. reduced mouth opening).
- Reduced neck mobility (e.g. rheumatoid arthritis).
- Airway pathology (e.g. tumours).
- Congenital conditions (e.g. Pierre Robin sequence, Marfan's syndrome).
- Normal anatomical variants (e.g. protruding teeth, small mouth, receding mandible).

Box 15.5 **Strategies for difficult intubation**

- Adjust position of patient: optimise head and neck position.
- Airway manoeuvres such as BURP (backward, upward and to the patient's right) may optimise the view by applying manipulation to the thyroid cartilage.
- Alternative laryngoscopes (e.g. straight blade, short handle).
- Intubation aids: gum elastic bougie or intubating stylet.
- Intubation through a laryngeal mask.
- Fibreoptic intubation.
- Surgical airway (e.g. cricothyroidotomy).

Remember that repeated attempts at intubation should be avoided. Patients die from failure to oxygenate rather than failure to intubate.

view of the vocal cords at laryngoscopy (Figure 15.13). It is, however, possible to have a good view of the cords at laryngoscopy but still have problems passing the endotracheal tube itself through the airway and past the vocal cords. Causes of difficult intubation can be found in Box 15.4 and a list of strategies for difficult intubation in Box 15.5.

Potential problems during intubation

Anatomical variations

Certain features of a patient's anatomy might make intubation difficult. In these cases it is essential to ensure adequate oxygenation rather than persisting with intubation attempts.

Physiological effects

Intubation is a potent stimulus to both the respiratory and cardiovascular systems. It must only be performed in the deeply unconscious patient. Respiratory effects include increased respiratory drive, laryngospasm and bronchospasm. Cardiovascular effects include tachycardia, hypertension and dysrhythmias.

Airway trauma

Dental and soft tissue damage can occur. This can be minimised by skilled intubation technique.

Gastric regurgitation

This may occur in any unconscious patient. It is advisable to have a functioning suction device to hand during intubation. Cricoid pressure may prevent passive regurgitation and subsequent aspiration.

Oesophageal intubation

This should be suspected when the oxygen saturation decreases despite an adequate supply of oxygen. A carbon dioxide (CO_2) detector attached to the tube indicates correct tracheal placement only if exhaled CO_2 persists after six ventilations. A look, listen and feel approach should be used to recognise oesophageal placement of the tube.

| Remember: if in any doubt take the tube out!

Cervical spine injury

Excessive movement of the head and neck must be avoided in this situation. The hard collar is removed whilst in-line manual stabilisation of the head and neck is performed by an assistant. The operator then intubates the airway.

Surgical airways

These are performed in an emergency when all possible manoeuvres to achieve effective ventilation and intubation have failed and the patient's oxygen saturations are falling. Percutaneous needle or surgical cricothyroidotomy are the immediate techniques of choice.

Percutaneous needle cricothyroidotomy

This involves puncturing the cricothyroid membrane (Figure 15.14) with a large-bore intravenous cannula attached to a syringe.

Surgical cricothyroidotomy

In this technique a blade is used to pierce the cricothyroid membrane. A small cuffed tracheal tube or purpose designed 4–6-mm cuffed cannula is then passed through the membrane.

Complications of surgical airways

- Trauma to surrounding structures.
- Haemorrhage.
- Surgical emphysema due to incorrect cannula placement.
- Pulmonary barotrauma: exhaled gases must be free to escape otherwise pressure builds up within the airway.

Cricoid pressure

This manoeuvre is performed to prevent gastric regurgitation with subsequent aspiration into the lungs in the anaesthetised patient. Digital pressure is applied to the cricoid cartilage pushing it backwards (Figure 15.15). This compresses the oesophagus between the posterior aspect of the cricoid and the vertebra behind. The cricoid is used since it is the only complete ring of cartilage in the larynx and trachea.

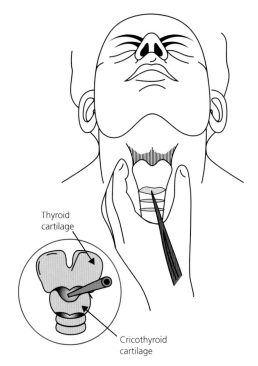

Thyroid cartilage

Cricothyroid cartilage

Figure 15.14 Cricothyroidotomy: the cannula is placed through the cricothyroid membrane. Redrawn from Beers MH (ed). (2006) *The Merck Manual of Diagnosis and Therapy*, 18th edition. Merck & Co.

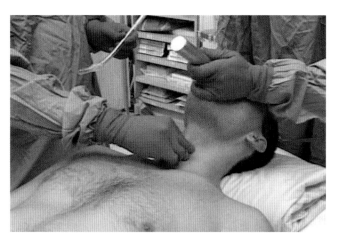

Figure 15.15 An assistant applies cricoid pressure whilst the operator performs laryngoscopy.

Technique for applying cricoid pressure

1 Identify the cricoid cartilage immediately below the thyroid cartilage.
2 Place the index finger against the cartilage in the midline, with the thumb and middle finger on either side. In an awake patient, moderate force (10 N) is applied before loss of consciousness; the force is then increased to 30 N until the cuff of the tracheal tube is inflated.
3 The assistant should release cricoid pressure only when clearly instructed to so by the person performing the intubation.

Handy hints/troubleshooting

- This needs to be learnt and practised in a safe environment rather than in an emergency situation.
- Always have a back-up plan. Know your difficult airway drill and always have senior help available.
- Maximise your first chance by optimal patient positioning.
- Don`t be afraid to ask for a bougie or different laryngoscope blade.
- 'If in doubt, take it out!'

Further reading

Benumof JL. (1991) Management of the difficult airway. *Anaesthesiology* **75**: 531–3.

Dolenska S, Dalal P, Taylor A. (2004) *Essentials of Airway Management.* Greenwich Medical Media, London.

Resuscitation Council UK. (2006) Airway management and ventilation. In: *Advanced Life Support Course-Provider Manual, 5th edn.* Resuscitation Council UK, London.

CHAPTER 16

Therapeutic: Ascitic Drain

Sharat Putta

Queen Elizabeth Hospital, Birmingham, UK

OVERVIEW

By the end of this chapter you should be able to:
- discuss the indications for insertion of an ascitic drain
- understand the anatomy relevant to insertion of the drain
- explain how to insert an ascitic drain
- understand the potential complications of this procedure.

Introduction

Ascitic drain or paracentesis refers to a procedure used to obtain fluid from the peritoneal cavity for diagnostic or therapeutic purposes.

Diagnostic paracentesis involves collection of 20–50 mL of fluid, for biochemical, cytological and microbiological investigation (discussed in Chapter 8).

Therapeutic paracentesis refers to the drainage of larger quantities of fluid to alleviate symptoms. Large-volume paracentesis (LVP) is a term used to denote the drainage of large quantities of ascitic fluid, typically greater than 5 L. Total paracentesis refers to complete drainage of all ascitic fluid. Volumes in excess of 15 L can be drained safely in a single session, with careful monitoring and intravenous fluid replacement.

Cirrhosis of the liver accounts for 80% of all causes of ascites (Box 16.1). It is therefore obvious that paracentesis is usually undertaken in this setting. As discussed later in this chapter, this is an exceedingly important issue, especially when considering therapeutic/large-volume paracentesis, due to the unique physiological and circulatory changes in cirrhosis and the impact of large-volume paracentesis on renal function and circulation.

Indications for therapeutic paracentesis

When large in volume or causing a tense abdomen, ascites leads to abdominal pain and mechanical effects such as respiratory compromise, early satiety, scrotal and leg swelling and frequently a poor quality of life.

Ascites from cirrhosis is often controlled with diuretic therapy, but a significant proportion of patients are either resistant

Box 16.1 **Causes of ascites**

Transudative ascites
- Cirrhosis of the liver
- Cardiac failure
- Nephrotic syndrome

Exudative ascites
- Cancer: gastric, ovarian, peritoneal carcinomatosis
- Tuberculous peritonitis
- Pancreatitis

Box 16.2 **Recommendations by the British Society of Gastroenterology for therapeutic paracentesis in cirrhosis**

- Therapeutic paracentesis is the first-line treatment for patients with large or refractory ascites. (Level of evidence: 1a; recommendation: A.)
- Paracentesis of 5 L of uncomplicated ascites should be followed by plasma expansion with a synthetic plasma expander and does not require volume expansion with albumin (Level of evidence: 2b; recommendation: B.)
- Large-volume paracentesis should be performed in a single session with volume expansion once paracentesis is complete, preferably using 8 g albumin/L of ascites removed (that is, 100 mL of 20% albumin/3 L ascites). (Level of evidence: 1b; recommendation: A.)

to or intolerant of diuretic therapy. Paracentesis enables effective symptom control in this group of patients in the short and long term, and is often required on a periodic basis. Therapeutic paracentesis is the first-line treatment for large or refractory ascites in the presence of cirrhosis (Box 16.2).

Ascites from malignant causes tends not to respond to diuretic therapy. Treatment of the underlying cause may lead to resolution of ascites, but a significant proportion of patients with malignant ascites have incurable metastatic disease and paracentesis is often required for palliation.

Contraindications

Although there are no absolute contraindications that preclude the procedure, caution needs to be exercised under the following circumstances.

ABC of Practical Procedures. Edited by T. Nutbeam and R. Daniels. © 2010 Blackwell Publishing, ISBN: 978-1-4051-8595-0.

Coagulopathy—There are no data to suggest absolute coagulation parameter cut-offs beyond which paracentensis should be avoided. It is prudent, however, to administer plasma coagulation factors immediately before the procedure under the following conditions:

- INR >2 or
- evidence of DIC or fibrinolysis.

Intravenous vitamin K is a simple and often overlooked intervention which if given in a timely fashion can lead to correction of INR before paracentesis.

Severe thrombocytopenia—Patients with platelet counts less than $20 \times 10^3/\mu L$ should receive an infusion of platelets before undergoing the procedure.

Abdominal wall cellulitis.

The following conditions can complicate the course of cirrhosis and caution needs to be exercised when paracentesis is being considered in these settings:

- subacute bacterial peritonitis (SBP)
- hepatorenal syndrome (HRS)
- hepatic encephalopathy (HE).

Haemodynamic changes in cirrhosis are unique, in that there is significant peripheral and splanchnic vasodilatation, with consequent decrease in effective circulating arterial volume leading to renal vasoconstriction and decreased renal perfusion. LVP in this setting leads to delayed hypovolemia. This typically occurs a few hours after the procedure and renal impairment can ensue as a result. SBP and pre-existing renal impairment increase the risk of renal failure following LVP. Hepatic encephalopathy can be precipitated or worsened by LVP.

In the presence of cirrhosis-related complications (HRS, SBP, HE) avoid LVP. Alternately consider limited paracentesis; drainage of between 2 and 5 L is often sufficient to relieve symptoms from large or tense ascites.

Landmarks and anatomy

The two commonest sites used for ascitic drainage are:

1 midline between the umbilicus and the pubic symphysis (through the linea alba)
2 5 cm superior and medial to the anterior superior iliac spines on either side, preferably on the left.

Epigastric blood vessels are usually located in the area between 4 and 8 cm from the midline. Staying away from this area will determine the safe zone of entry into the anterior abdominal wall. The midline below the umbilicus is the safest avascular zone. However, one has to exercise caution to ensure that the urinary bladder is empty, as the bladder could easily be punctured if it is full. A simple routine would be to ask the patient to void before insertion of the peritoneal catheter. Alternatively a bedside bladder scan could be performed to ensure that the bladder is empty. Avoid areas of scar tissue as small bowel is often adherent to abdominal scars and can easily be punctured. Avoid areas containing prominent abdominal wall veins.

Role of ultrasound

Paracentesis is often an easy procedure to undertake in the presence of gross ascites and a non-obese subject. Even in the presence of significant ascites, paracentesis can sometimes be difficult in obese individuals and patients who have undergone multiple abdominal operations (as fluid can be loculated and small bowel may be adherent to the abdominal wall with consequent risk of hollow viscus perforation). Ultrasound can be useful in determining the site for entry, confirming the presence and the depth of the pocket of fluid and in avoiding a distended urinary bladder (if using the midline approach) or small bowel adhesions below the entry point.

Step-by-step guide: insertion of ascitic drain

- **Give a full explanation to the patient in simple terms and ensure they consent to the procedure.**
- **Set up your trolley (Box 16.3 and Figure 16.1).**
- **Prepare your trolley as a sterile field. Wear a plastic disposable apron and non-sterile gloves, and take alcohol hand rub with you.**

Box 16.3 **Equipment for insertion of ascitic drain**

- Rocket catheter/drain *or* the Bonanno™ suprapubic catheter. Both of these catheters consist of a straight metal trocar, which serves as a core for a plastic tube with a curved end that is kept straight while the trocar is inside. The Bonanno™ catheter has a small flat plate on one end that can be taped or sutured to the skin.
- 25G and 21G needles.
- Dressing set containing sterile drapes and sterile gloves.
- Chlorhexidine solution for cleansing.
- Transparent adhesive dressing.
- Catheter drainage bag.

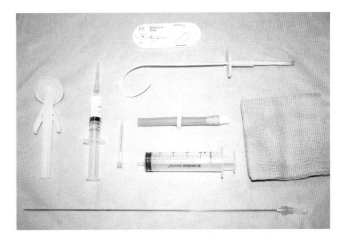

Figure 16.1 The equipment required for insertion of ascitic drain.

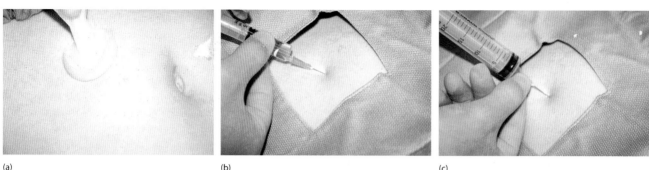

(a)   (b)   (c)

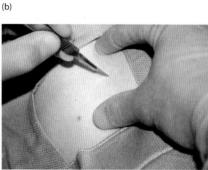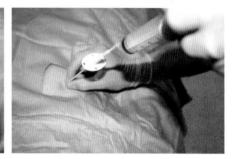

(d)   (e)   (f)

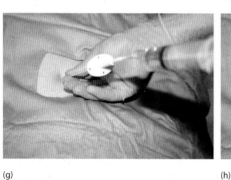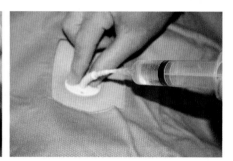

(g)   (h)   (i)

(j)

Figure 16.2 Step-by-step guide: insertion of ascitic drain. (a) Cleaning the area (2% chlorhexidine in 70% alcohol). (b) Infiltration of local anaesthetic. (c) Aspirating whilst advancing the green needle. (d) Successful aspiration of peritoneal fluid (the needle is not advanced any further). (e) Making a small incision. (f) Aspirating whilst advancing the catheter. (g) Flashback of peritoneal fluid. (h) Sliding the catheter over the needle. (i) Checking the position of the catheter once fully advanced (can still aspirate peritoneal fluid). (j) Catheter sutured in position.

1 Identify the catheter insertion site, preferably in the left lower abdomen.
2 Wash hands thoroughly and don a sterile gown and gloves, considering also personal protective equipment.
3 Cleanse with antiseptic solution (e.g. 2% chlorhexidine in 70% alcohol) and drape the area with sterile towels (Figure 16.2a).
4 Take 10 mL of 1 or 2% lidocaine in a 10-mL syringe. Using a 25G orange needle, raise a small skin bleb around the skin entry site.

5 Use a 21G green needle to inoculate lidocaine into the skin, subcutaneous tissues, muscles and parietal peritoneum. Maintain the needle perpendicular to the abdominal wall at all times (Figure 16.2b,c).
6 Note the depth at which the peritoneum is entered (when ascites can be aspirated back into the syringe). You must always be able to drain ascites with the green needle and syringe before inserting the peritoneal catheter and note the depth at which peritoneum is reached (Figure 16.2d).

7 Use a scalpel blade to make a small nick in the skin to allow for easy catheter access (Figure 16.2e). Insert the catheter perpendicular to the selected entry point (Figure 16.2f). Insert slowly in increments of 5 mm to minimise the risk of inadvertent vascular entry. Continuously apply suction to the syringe as the needle is advanced.

8 Sudden loss of resistance is felt when you enter the peritoneal cavity and ascitic fluid can be aspirated into the syringe (Figure 16.2g). At this point, advance the catheter a further 5 mm into the peritoneal cavity. Avoid advancing the catheter any deeper.

9 Use one hand to firmly hold the trocar and syringe in place to prevent the trocar from entering further into the peritoneal cavity. Use the other hand to advance the plastic catheter over the trocar all the way into the peritoneal cavity (Figure 16.2h). Resistance should not be felt while the catheter is advanced. Resistance could mean that the catheter has been misplaced. If resistance is felt withdraw the catheter completely and reattempt the procedure.

10 Remove the trocar once the plastic catheter is completely inserted, and attach the three-way stopcock and a catheter bag. Ascitic fluid should drain completely within 4–6 hours through gravity.

11 Secure the drain with sutures or an appropriate purpose-made dressing (Figure 16.2j). Use the 'Z' technique, to avoid leakage of ascites post procedure. This involves stretching the skin a couple of centimetres in any direction over the deep abdominal wall. The catheter is then inserted into the peritoneum. Upon releasing the skin a Z tract is created in that the entry points in the skin and the peritoneum are not directly against each other. Although there is little evidence to back up this theory, it is believed to minimise the risk of persistent leak from the puncture site.

Complications

Paracentesis is a very safe procedure, and complications are rare if simple precautions are exercised.

Immediate complications
- Abdominal wall haematoma.
- Haemoperitoneum. This rare complication can result from trauma to a major blood vessel or intraabdominal varices at the time of insertion of the peritoneal catheter.
- Hollow viscus perforation. Simple precautions like careful selection of the entry site with attention to avoiding scars and obvious abdominal wall veins should minimise the risk of hollow viscus perforation or bleeding. Alternately an ultrasound scan can be performed before the procedure to select the entry site.
- Liver or splenic laceration.
- Catheter laceration and loss in abdominal cavity.

- Ascitic leakage. This is one of the commonest complications following paracentesis. Ascites can leak from the puncture site, often for several days after the procedure. Ostomy bags can be used around the puncture site to keep the leak contained until it eventually ceases. Several hundred mL of fluid can drain into the bag every day and some patients find this advantageous in controlling their ascites. Alternatively a single suture can be applied to close the puncture site.
- Failed paracentesis.

Late complications
- Postparacentesis hypovolemia and hypotension. This is the most important physiological phenomenon that frequently complicates paracentesis, especially in the setting of cirrhosis of the liver. As discussed earlier, renal failure can occur as a result of the haemodynamic changes following paracentesis. The risk of renal failure is especially increased in patients with spontaneous bacterial peritonitis or pre-existing renal impairment. Administration of human albumin corrects intravascular hypovolemia and is the single most important therapeutic intervention that could prevent renal failure following large-volume paracentesis in cirrhosis. Frequent monitoring of vital signs following paracentesis is important in identifying haemodynamic changes and correcting them appropriately.
- Hyponatraemia.
- Hepatorenal syndrome.

Handy hints/troubleshooting

- Always check the clotting: a recent INR and platelet count should be assessed before starting the procedure.
- In obese patients the 21G green needle may not be long enough to reach the peritoneum. Use a needle from a green cannula (18G) which is much longer than a standard 21G needle.
- Ensure the drain is well secured.
- Ensure there is a clear plan documented in the notes regarding drainage volumes and replacement fluids.

Further reading

Gines P, Tito L, Arroyo V et al. (1988) Randomized study of therapeutic paracentesis with and without intravenous albumin in cirrhosis. *Gastroenterology* 94: 1493–502.

Moore KP, Aithal GP. (2006) Guidelines on the management of ascites in cirrhosis. *Gut* 55: 1–12.

Panos MZ, Moore K, Vlavianos P et al. (1990) Single total paracentesis for tense ascites: sequential haemodynamic changes and right atrial size. *Hepatology* 11: 667.

Saber AA, Meslemani AM. (2004) Safety zones for anterior abdominal wall entry during laparoscopy: a ct scan mapping of epigastric vessels. *Ann Surg* 239(2): 182–5.

CHAPTER 17

Therapeutic: Chest Drain

Nicola Sinden

West Midlands Rotation, Birmingham, UK

OVERVIEW

By the end of this chapter you should be able to:
- understand the principles of managing a pneumothorax
- understand the indications and contraindications for insertion of a chest drain
- identify and understand the relevant anatomy
- be aware of different types of chest drains
- describe the procedure of performing a Seldinger and surgical chest drain
- identify and manage a tension pneumothorax.

Management of pneumothorax

A pneumothorax is defined as air in the pleural space (Figure 17.1). Pneumothorax may be primary, with no existing lung disease, or secondary to an underlying disease. Examples of secondary pneumothorax include: traumatic (Figure 17.2), iatrogenic or a disease process such as asthma.

According to current British Thoracic Society (BTS) guidelines, a primary pneumothorax may not require any treatment if the patient is not breathless and the pneumothorax is small (rim of air <2 cm). If treatment is indicated, then the guidelines state that aspiration should be attempted first, and a second attempt should be considered if the first is unsuccessful. If aspiration is unsuccessful or repeated aspiration becomes necessary then an intercostal drain should be inserted. However, in clinical practice, intercostal drain insertion may be used as the initial treatment in a patient presenting with a large primary pneumothorax.

A secondary pneumothorax is usually treated initially with an intercostal drain unless the patient is not breathless, is under 50 years of age and the pneumothorax is small (rim of air <2 cm).

Indications for intercostal drain insertion
- Primary pneumothorax following unsuccessful aspiration.
- Secondary pneumothorax.
- Tension pneumothorax following needle decompression (see Box 17.3).

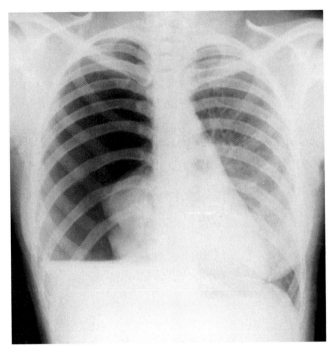

Figure 17.1 A large right-sided pneumothorax.

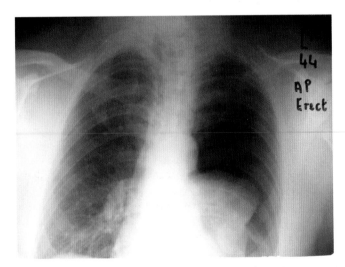

Figure 17.2 A traumatic pneumothorax.

ABC of Practical Procedures. Edited by T. Nutbeam and R. Daniels. © 2010
Blackwell Publishing, ISBN: 978-1-4051-8595-0.

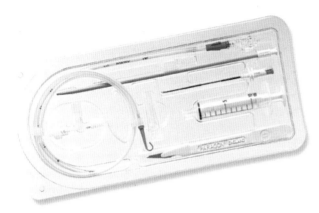

Figure 17.3 A Seldinger chest drain.

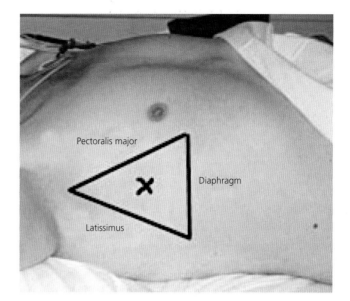

Figure 17.4 The 'triangle of safety'.

- Pneumothorax in a ventilated patient.
- Empyema and complicated parapneumonic effusions (pleural fluid pH<7.2).
- Haemothorax.
- Malignant pleural effusion for symptomatic relief (and for performing pleurodesis).
- Large pleural effusions of other aetiology.

Contraindications to intercostal drain insertion
- Inexperience with technique.
- Refusal by a competent patient.
- Deranged INR/platelets (stop warfarin and correct any coagulopathy).
- Lung adherent to the chest wall.
- Drainage of a post-pneumonectomy space should only be carried out after consultation with a cardiothoracic surgeon.

Types of chest drain

Trocar chest drains consist of a plastic drain with a radio-opaque stripe along their length surrounding a metal rod with a sharp end. They are available in a variety of sizes.

Seldinger (Figure 17.3) chest drains are usually smaller drains which are inserted by advancing the drain over a guidewire. Studies have shown that smaller chest drains (10–14F) are often as effective as larger-bore drains and are better tolerated by patients.

Large-bore drains are recommended for acute haemothorax to monitor blood loss and may also be necessary if a pneumothorax has failed to resolve despite a smaller drain.

Anatomy and positioning of patient

Chest drains should be inserted within the 'triangle of safety' which has the following borders (see Figure 17.4):
- anteriorly – anterior axillary line, lateral border of pectoralis major
- posteriorly – anterior border of latissimus dorsi
- inferiorly – at the level of the nipple.

Ideally the patient should be positioned on the bed at 45° with their arm held behind their head to expose the axillary area. Alternatively, the patient could be sitting forwards and leaning over a table.

Box 17.1 **Equipment for insertion of a Seldinger chest drain**

- Dressing pack and solution (we recommend 2% chlorhexidine/70% isopropyl alcohol) for cleansing of the skin
- Sterile gloves
- Sterile drapes
- Gauze
- 1 or 2% lidocaine
- 10-mL syringe for local anaesthetic
- One blue needle
- One green needle
- Scalpel
- Seldinger chest drain pack
- Chest drain bottle and tubing
- Sterile water for drain bottle
- Suture (e.g. size 1 silk)
- Dressing for site of drain insertion

Ultrasound guidance
Recent research regarding the morbidity and mortality of chest drain insertion strongly recommends insertion of chest drains under ultrasound guidance. The ultrasound training required for this is beyond the scope of this text, but healthcare professionals who intend to perform this procedure should familiarise themselves with this.

Step-by-step guide: insertion of a Seldinger chest drain

- **Give a full explanation to the patient in simple terms and ensure they consent to the procedure.**
- **Set up your trolley (Box 17.1 and Figure 17.5).**
- **Prepare your trolley as a sterile field. Wear a plastic disposable apron and sterile gloves, and take alcohol hand rub with you.**

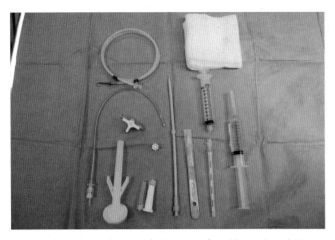

Figure 17.5 Equipment required for insertion of a Seldinger chest drain.

1 Verify the correct side by clinical examination, review of the CXR and ultrasound.

2 Consider premedication with a benzodiazepine or opioid to reduce patient distress but beware of respiratory depression.

3 Use a strict aseptic technique. Wear sterile gloves and gown; consider also a facemask with visor. Prepare the skin with antiseptic solution and allow to dry. Apply a sterile drape (Figure 17.6a).

4 Infiltrate the skin with local anaesthetic using a blue (23G) or orange (25G) needle (Figure 17.6b). Then use a green needle (21G) to infiltrate deeper and anaesthetise the parietal pleura (Figure 17.6c). The needle should be inserted just above the upper border of the rib to avoid the intercostal neurovascular bundle. Always aspirate before injecting local anaesthetic to ensure that you are not in a blood vessel. Verify that the site is correct by aspirating fluid or air with a green needle (21G). If this is not possible do not proceed with drain insertion and consider image-guided drainage.

5 Whilst giving the local anaesthetic time to work, prepare the Seldinger chest drain pack. This will usually consist of an introducer needle, 10-mL syringe, guidewire, dilator(s) and drain. Also prepare the underwater seal bottle by filling the bottle with sterile water up to the marked point on the bottle and by attaching the tubing. Different types of bottle exist so it is important to familiarise yourself with the equipment available at your hospital.

6 Attach the introducer needle to the 10-mL syringe. Insert the needle through the area of skin and pleura which has been anaesthetised and aim just above the upper border of the rib (Figure 17.6d). Confirm correct positioning within the pleural space by aspirating fluid or air. Once in the pleural space do not advance the introducer needle further.

7 Remove the 10-mL syringe from the end of the introducer needle and place your sterile-gloved thumb over the end to prevent air entering the pleural cavity.

8 Smoothly insert the guidewire through the introducer needle (Figure 17.6e). There should not be any resistance felt if positioning is correct.

9 Using the scalpel make a small 'stab' incision at the base of the needle.

10 Remove the introducer needle whilst keeping hold of the guidewire.

11 Take the dilator and slide it over the guidewire to enlarge the tract (Figure 17.6f). Ensure that you keep hold of the end of the guidewire whilst inserting the dilator. The dilator only needs to be inserted a short distance into the pleural cavity. The depth can be judged by the size of the initial needle used to aspirate fluid or air. For larger chest drains there may be more than one dilator in the pack. In this case, start with the smallest dilator and progress to the largest.

12 Slide the drain over the guidewire and into the pleural cavity (Figure 17.6g). Once the drain is in the pleural cavity the guidewire can be removed. The three-way tap should be kept covered (Figure 17.6h) or in the closed position until the drain is attached to the underwater seal bottle (Figure 17.6i).

13 Place a suture through the skin adjacent to the drain and tie the suture into the skin and subsequently around the drain until it is secure (Figure 17.6j).

14 Finally place a dressing over the drain insertion site. If the drain is correctly positioned it should swing with respiration and drain fluid or air.

15 Ask for a CXR after the procedure and ensure that adequate analgesia is prescribed.

Step-by-step guide: insertion of a trocar chest drain

1 Carry out steps **1** to **4** as described above (Figure 17.7a). Your trolley should be set up with the equipment listed in Box 17.2. Prepare the underwater seal bottle by filling the bottle with sterile water up to the marked point on the bottle and by attaching the tubing.

2 Make a skin incision parallel to the rib slightly larger in size to the diameter of the tube being inserted (Figure 17.7b).

3 Put a horizontal mattress suture (see Figure 17.8) across the incision to assist with later closure.

4 Perform blunt dissection using blunt forceps (e.g. Spencer Wells) (see Figure 17.9).

5 Insert the forceps through the skin incision and separate the muscle fibres by opening and withdrawing the forceps (Figure 17.7c). Do not close the forceps as this may cause damage. Continue blunt dissection through the intercostal muscles and parietal pleura. The tract should be explored with a finger to ensure that there are no underlying organs that may be damaged by drain insertion (including the lung itself!) (Figure 17.7d).

6 Remove the trocar from the drain. *The trocar should never be used to insert a chest drain.* Hold the end of the chest drain with blunt forceps and guide the drain into the pleural cavity. Excessive force should not be needed. If resistance is felt then further blunt dissection is required. Some manufacturers provide an introducer to aid with insertion of the drain (Figure 17.7e). The tip of the drain should be aimed apically for a pneumothorax and basally for an effusion, but functioning tubes should not be repositioned purely because of their radiological position.

7 Connect the drain to the underwater seal bottle.

8 Place a suture through the skin adjacent to the drain and tie the suture into the skin and subsequently around the drain until it is secure (Figure 17.7f,g).

9 Carry out steps **14** to **15** as described above. Figure 17.10 shows a large intercostal drain in situ.

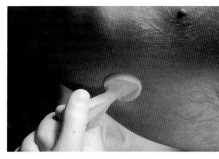

(a)

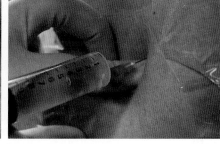

(b)

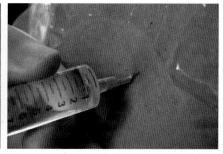

(c)

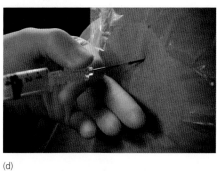

(d)

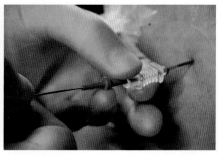

(e)

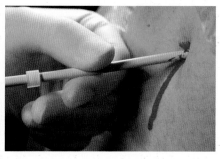

(f)

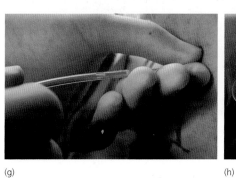

(g)

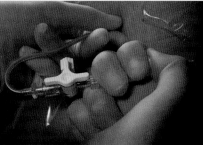

(h)

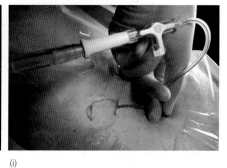

(i)

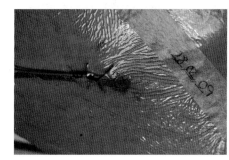

(j)

Figure 17.6 Step-by-step guide: Seldinger technique. (a) Sterilising the area with 2% chlorhexidine in 70% isopropyl alcohol. (b) Infiltrating local anaesthetic with blue needle. (c) Infiltrating local anaesthetic with green needle. (d) Inserting the trocar needle. (e) Inserting the Seldinger wire. (f) Dilating over the wire. (g) Inserting the drain. (h) Connecting the three-way tap (ensuring not open to air). (i) Connecting the drain to the underwater seal. (j) The drain sutured in position and dressed.

Complications following intercostal drain insertion

- Pain (prescribe simple and/or opioid analgesia).
- Infection.
- Poor position of drain: may need withdrawing slightly.
- Blockage of drain: may require flush with 10 mL sterile saline.
- Organ damage: do not insert the sharp trocar into the pleural cavity.
- Bleeding: stop warfarin before insertion and correct any coagulopathy.
- Surgical emphysema may occur with pneumothorax.

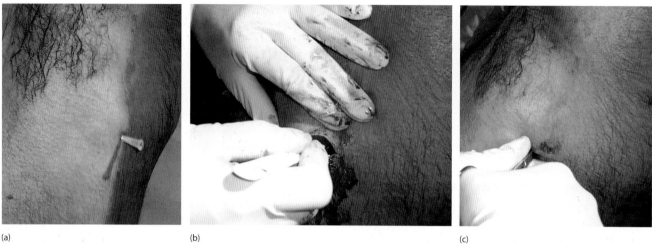

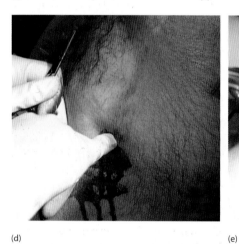

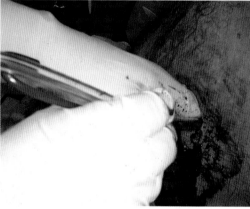

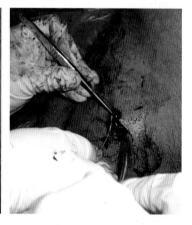

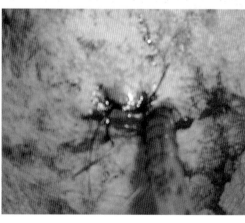

Figure 17.7 Step-by-step guide: trocar technique. (a) The insertion site prepped, local anaesthetic infiltrated and site marked with green needle. (b) Initial incision. (c) Blunt dissection using forceps. (d) Blunt dissection with finger. (e) Insertion of large drain using introducer. (f) Suturing the drain in position. (g) The drain secured in position.

- Re-expansion pulmonary oedema. Following drainage of a large effusion or pneumothorax, negative intrathoracic pressure caused by rapid re-expansion of the lung may cause non-cardiogenic pulmonary oedema.

Management of intercostal drains

- Patients with chest drains should be managed on specialist wards by trained staff. Chest drain charts should be kept which document whether the drain is swinging or bubbling, and the volume of fluid drained.
- Keep the bottle upright and below the level of the insertion site.
- A bubbling chest drain should never be clamped.
- When a drain is inserted for a pleural effusion, the drain should be clamped for 1 hour after draining 1 litre of fluid to reduce the risk of re-expansion pulmonary oedema.

- Dressing pack and solution (we recommend 2% chlorhexidine/70% isopropyl alcohol) for cleansing of the skin
- Sterile gloves
- Sterile drapes
- Gauze
- 1 or 2% lidocaine
- 10-mL syringe for local anaesthetic
- One blue needle
- One green needle
- Scalpel
- Forceps for blunt dissection e.g. Spencer Wells
- Trocar chest drain
- Chest drain bottle and tubing
- Sterile water for drain bottle
- Suture (e.g. size 1 silk)
- Dressing for site of drain insertion

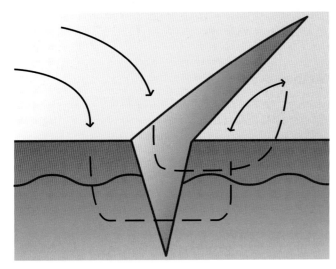

Figure 17.8 A horizontal mattress suture.

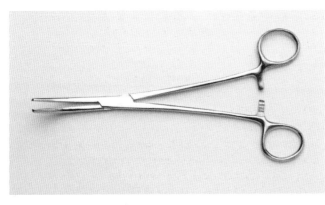

Figure 17.9 Spencer Wells forceps.

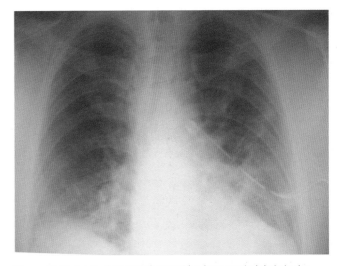

Figure 17.10 Resolved pneumothorax with a large surgical drain in situ.

- If a pneumothorax fails to resolve after 48 hours, refer to a respiratory physician and consider adding high-volume/low-pressure suction (e.g. 2.5–5 kPa). You may also consider inserting a bigger drain. Discuss with the cardiothoracic surgeons if a pneumothorax fails to resolve after 3–5 days.
- If a drain stops swinging, it may be blocked, kinked or malpositioned. A blocked drain may be unblocked with a flush of 10 mL of sterile saline. A non-functioning drain should be removed.

Removal of intercostal drains

- Following a pneumothorax, the chest drain can be removed when the drain has stopped bubbling for 24 hours and a CXR confirms re-expansion of the lung.
- Following a pleural effusion, the chest drain can be removed when the CXR shows resolution of the effusion. Drain output will usually be less than 100 mL per day.
- To remove a chest drain, firstly cut the sutures which are holding the drain in the skin. Ask the patient to hold their breath in expiration or perform a Valsalva manoeuvre and remove the chest drain. A suture will be required after removal of larger drains. A mattress suture may have been previously placed for this purpose. Apply a dressing and perform a CXR after drain removal.

Discharge and follow-up of patients with pneumothorax

- Patients with a pneumothorax who are discharged without active intervention should be advised to return in 2 weeks' time for a follow-up CXR.
- Patients should be advised to avoid air travel until 6 weeks following resolution of the pneumothorax.
- Scuba diving should be permanently avoided by patients who have had a pneumothorax unless they undergo bilateral surgical pleurectomy.
- All patients should be given advice to return immediately should they experience worsening breathlessness.

Tension pneumothorax

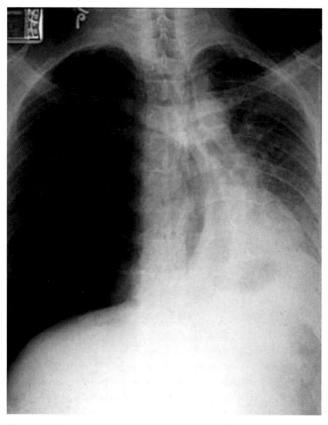

Figure 17.11 A tension pneumothorax: complete collapse of the right lung can be seen with the mediastinum forced over to the patient's left.

Box 17.3 **Management of a tension pneumothorax**

A tension pneumothorax (Figure 17.11) is a life-threatening emergency that requires prompt diagnosis and treatment. It occurs when gas accumulating in the pleural space cannot escape, most commonly due to trauma (e.g. penetrating stab wound), or arising from positive-pressure ventilation.

Features:
• acute respiratory distress
• absent breath sounds on affected side
• tachycardia and hypotension.
Signs which may be harder to illicit include tracheal deviation away from affected side, distension of neck veins and hyperresonance over affected side.

If tension pneumothorax is present, a cannula of adequate length should be promptly inserted into the second intercostal space in the midclavicular line and left in place until a functioning intercostal drain is inserted.

A tension pneumothorax is a clinical diagnosis and should never be imaged (it needs urgent treatment).

Learning points

• Smaller chest drains (10–14F) are usually effective and well tolerated by patients.
• Chest drains should be inserted within the 'triangle of safety.'
• Never use excessive force when inserting a chest drain.
• Never use the Trocar rod to insert the chest drain.
• Never clamp a bubbling chest drain.

Handy hints/troubleshooting

• Take time to explain the procedure thoroughly to the patient, and talk them through it if appropriate.
• Positioning the patient in a comfortable position is vital – they are going to be there for some time.
• If you are sedating the patient you should have two medical practitioners, one doing the procedure and one responsible for sedation and monitoring.
• Use plenty of local anaesthetic – the maximum dose of 1% lidocaine is approximately 20 mL for an average-sized adult.
• Stitching in the chest drain securely is vital – they are notorious for falling out. This is not only annoying, but can also be very dangerous.
• Remember to order (and look at) the post-procedure chest X-ray and document the result.

Further reading

Antunes G, Neville E, Duffy J, Ali N. (2003) BTS Guidelines for the Management of Malignant Pleural Effusions. *Thorax* 58 (Suppl II): ii29–ii38.

Chapman S, Robinson G, Stradling J, West S. (2005) *Oxford Handbook of Respiratory Medicine.* Oxford University Press, Oxford.

Davies CWH, Gleeson FV, Davies RJO. (2003) BTS Guidelines for the Management of Pleural Infection. *Thorax* 58 (Suppl II): ii18–ii28.

Henry M, Arnold T, Harvey J. (2003) BTS Guidelines for the Management of Spontaneous Pneumothorax. *Thorax* 58 (Suppl II): ii39–ii52.

Laws D, Neville E, Duffy J. (2003) BTS Guidelines for the Insertion of a Chest Drain. *Thorax* 58 (Suppl II): ii53–ii59.

Maskell NA, Butland RJA. (2003) BTS Guidelines for the Investigation of a Unilateral Pleural Effusion in Adults. *Thorax* 58 (suppl II): ii8–ii17.

National Patient Safety Agency. (2008) *Rapid Response Report: Risks of Chest Drain Insertion.* National Patient Safety Agency, London.

CHAPTER 18

Monitoring: Urinary Catheterisation

Adam Low[1] and Michael Foster[2]

[1]*University Hospital Birmingham, Birmingham, UK*
[2]*Heart of England NHS Foundation Trust, Good Hope Hospital, Birmingham, UK*

OVERVIEW

By the end of this chapter you should be able to:
- understand the indications and contraindications for insertion of a urinary catheter
- identify and understand the relevant anatomy
- be aware of different types of urinary catheter
- describe the procedure of performing a urethral and suprapubic catheterisation
- understand the complications of urethral and suprapubic catheterisation.

Introduction

Urinary catheterisation is a relatively simple practical procedure to master and gets easier with practice. It is important to familiarise yourself with the catheter packs used in your hospital and the catheter types available in your clinical area. Remember to take a chaperone with you and always document this in the notes. Follow your hospital's infection control procedures.

Urethral catheterisation

Indications
- Acute urinary retention.
- To monitor fluid balance, for example in septic and shocked patients.
- Epidural/spinal anaesthesia or in sedated patients.
- Intraoperatively.
- Deeply unconscious patient – for example tricyclic antidepressant overdose.
- To manage urinary incontinence, for example in elderly patients who are immobile and incontinent.
- To irrigate the bladder in cases of profuse haematuria.
- Intravesical drug therapy, for example to administer chemotherapy in bladder carcinoma.

ABC of Practical Procedures. Edited by T. Nutbeam and R. Daniels. © 2010
Blackwell Publishing, ISBN: 978-1-4051-8595-0.

Contraindications
- Pelvic trauma – check for blood at the urethral meatus and perform a digital rectal examination for a high riding prostate. This would suggest a urethral tear and catheterisation may cause additional trauma.
- A relative contraindication is a known urethral stricture which would make urethral catheterisation difficult. A specialist urology opinion should be sought.

Urogenital anatomy

The differences in male and female urogentital anatomy are illustrated in Figures 18.1 and 18.2. The main difference is in urethral length; the male urethra is 18–20 cm long and the female is just

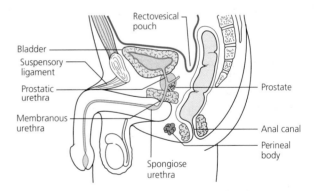

Figure 18.1 A sagittal section through the male pelvis. (From Faiz O, Moffat D. (2006) *Anatomy at a Glance*, 2nd edn. Blackwell Publishing, Oxford, with permission.)

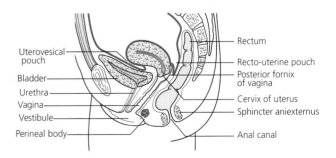

Figure 18.2 A sagittal section through the female pelvis. (From Faiz O, Moffat D. (2006) *Anatomy at a Glance*, 2nd edn. Blackwell Publishing, Oxford, with permission.)

4 cm long. The male urethra passes through the prostate gland which may make catheterisation more difficult if the prostate is enlarged.

Catheter types

There are different catheters for males and females due to the differing length of urethra. A male catheter can be used in female patients. Foley catheters have a balloon to keep them in place. Originally invented by Fredrick Foley, the intention for use was to achieve haemostasis and so there were different sizes of balloon available – 10, 20 and 30 mL. You will most commonly use the 10-mL balloon for urinary catheterisation where the balloon acts to keep the catheter in situ. Do not inflate the balloon with air as the balloon will float and may cause irritation. Use sterile water (saline can crystallise making it difficult to deflate the balloon). Most catheters come with a prefilled syringe.

Catheters also vary in external diameter which is measured in charrière (Ch); 1 charrière = 0.33 mm. 12, 14 and 16 Ch are most commonly available. A larger diameter will allow quicker drainage. Larger sizes should be used if clots or postoperative debris are present in the bladder. In general, use a size 14 Ch.

Catheters are made from different materials depending upon how long they are intended to be in situ.

Short-term catheters

- Plain latex: 7 days maximum, ideally 3 days. The latex gradually absorbs fluid, increasing its external and internal diameter, reducing urine flow and causing increasing discomfort.
- Plastic/polyvinyl chloride: used in theatre or for intermittent self-catheterisation. They are prone to bacterial contamination. They are a harder material, less flexible and can be uncomfortable.

Mid-term catheters

- Polytetrafluoroethylene: covers latex making the catheter smoother and less irritating. There is less fluid absorption but the polytetrafluoroethylene wears off after 3–4 weeks.

Long-term catheters

- Latex coated. This can be either with hydrogel, polymer hydromer or silicone elastomer, making the catheter smoother, reducing risk of bacterial colonisation and preventing fluid absorption. The catheter can be kept in for up to 12 weeks.
- Silicone: used in patients allergic to latex. Silicone is a less flexible material and the sterile water in the balloon diffuses gradually out into the bladder: a note should be made to check and top up the balloon after 6 weeks. The thickness of the silicone is less than latex-based catheters. Therefore they have a larger internal diameter with subsequent better drainage to comparable Ch sizes of latex catheter. Again, they can be kept in for up to 12 weeks.

Specialist catheters

- Three-way catheters: these have a third port that allows irrigation to run into the bladder. The catheter itself has a large diameter to allow blood and debris to pass into the drainage bag.
- Coude/Tiemann catheters: have a 45° bend at the tip allowing easier passage through an enlarged prostate.

- Council tip catheters: have a small hole in the end to allow passage over a guidewire.

> **Box 18.1 Equipment for insertion of a urinary catheter**
>
> Most hospitals stock catheter packs which contain most of the things you will need. While assembling your trolley you will need the following:
> - two pairs of sterile gloves
> - incontinence pad to place underneath the patient
> - lubricant – commonly contains lidocaine 2% and chlorhexidine 0.25% alongside lubricating gel
> - catheter pack + 10-mL syringe (normally prefilled)
> - cleaning solution (saline or chlorhexidine-based cleaning solution)
> - catheter: keep the stickers from the packaging to stick into the notes
> - catheter bag (depending on indication or need: can be a leg-bag that attaches to the patient's inside leg, an hourly bag for accurate measurement or 4-hourly bag)
> - catheter stand.

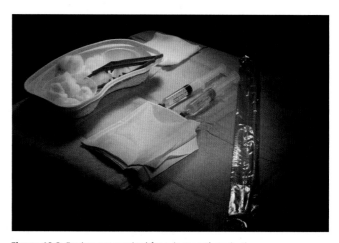

Figure 18.3 Equipment required for urinary catheterisation.

Step-by-step guide: urinary catheterisation

- **Give a full explanation to the patient in simple terms and ensure they consent to the procedure.**
- **Set up your trolley (Box 18.1 and Figure 18.3)**
- **Prepare your trolley as a sterile field. Wear a plastic disposable apron and sterile gloves, and take alcohol hand rub with you.**

1 Set up your sterile field and put on sterile gloves.
2 Position the patient lying supine on an incontinence pad and maintain their dignity at all times (Figure 18.4a). Obese or pregnant women may need to be positioned differently with knees bent to a greater extent or in the left lateral position if heavily pregnant.
3 Clean around the urethral meatus with cleaning solution (normal saline is acceptable) using a one wipe technique, cleaning downwards then disposing of the gauze (do not place the dirty gauze back into your sterile field) (Figure 18.4b). Repeat this until satisfied the area is clean. In females you will need to

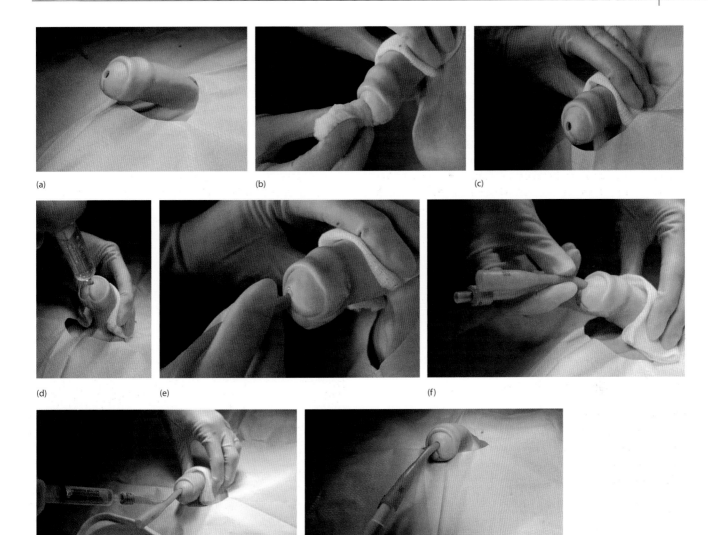

(a)   (b)   (c)

(d)   (e)   (f)

(g)   (h)

Figure 18.4 Step-by-step guide: urinary catheterisation. (a) Aperture drape around penis. (b) Cleaning the meatus. (c) Holding penis with gauze to maintain sterility. (d) Insertion of lubricant gel into the urethra. (e) Insertion of catheter. (f) Catheter fully inserted. (g) Filling the balloon with sterile water. (h) The catheter connected to collection bag.

separate the labia with your non-dominant hand; in males hold the shaft of the penis with some gauze (Figure 18.4c) and retract the foreskin if necessary.

4 Remove your first pair of gloves, clean your hands with alcohol gel and put on the second pair of sterile gloves.

5 Remove the catheter from its plastic covering and place it in the provided kidney dish from the catheter pack.

6 Take the sterile white sheet from the catheter pack and tear a small hole in the middle fold (unless already fenestrated). Place this across the patient with the hole over the genital area giving access to the urethra.

7 Insert lubricant into the urethra (Figure 18.4d). In males hold the penis at 90° and squeeze the tip of the penis gently to keep the gel in. In theory you should allow 5 minutes for preparations with local anaesthetics in them to have full effect. This, however, is rarely practical.

8 Feed the tip of the catheter into the urethra and up to the bifurcation of the catheter (Figure 18.4e,f). In males position the penis at 45° to straighten the urethra. Encourage the patient to take slow deep breaths in and out, especially in males as you pass through the prostate. If you are having difficulty, change the angle at which you are holding the penis and gently try a twisting motion – this may help you to get past the prostate. Remember, you may not see urine draining straight away as there may be some lubricant temporarily blocking the catheter.

9 Once urine is draining, fill the balloon up with 10 mL of sterile water (Figure 18.4g).

10 Do not pull the catheter back on the balloon – this can be uncomfortable. Allow gravity to do the work for you!

11 Attach the appropriate catheter bag (Figure 18.4h). Before you do so, do you need to send a urine sample, for example as part of a septic screen? If so, remember to document on the lab request form that it is a catheter sample of urine (CSU). Attach the bag to the stand.

12 In uncircumcised males, make sure that you replace the foreskin back over the glans penis to prevent paraphimosis (and document this in the notes).

13 Make sure the patient is comfortable, clean and dry before leaving the bedside.

14 Dispose of all your waste from the procedure in yellow clinical waste bags.

15 Document the procedure in the notes including your name, grade, date, time, name of your chaperone, indications for catheterisation, type of catheter inserted, volume of sterile water inserted into the balloon, date that the catheter should be reviewed and date when it should be removed or changed.

Potential complications (listed early to late)

- Urethral trauma: reduced by using adequate lubricant.
- Haematuria: this should settle. If this starts after a catheter has been in situ for some time it may require further investigation.
- Urinary tract infections and pyelonephritis: treat with oral/IV antibiotics according to microbiology advice and consider removing the catheter. Always send a 'catheter sample of urine' (CSU). Note that the presence of bacteria in the urine alone does NOT confirm a UTI.
- Debris and stone formation leading to catheter blockage – flush the catheter and consider removing or changing it.
- Traumatic hypospadias in long-term male catheters – always examine for this, especially in the community. The patient may then require suprapubic catheterisation.

Removal of catheter

A trial without catheter (TWOC) should generally be undertaken in the morning so that if recatheterisation is required it can be done during normal working hours.

1 Check in the notes how much water was inserted into the balloon.

2 Clean around the urethral meatus and catheter itself.

3 Use a 10-mL syringe to deflate the balloon and ensure the same volume comes out as was inserted.

4 Ask the patient to relax and take some slow breaths; this relaxes the pelvic floor muscles.

5 Remove the catheter as gently as possible – the deflated balloon may cause discomfort in male patients as it passes through the prostate so warn patients of this.

6 Dispose of the catheter and bag in clinical waste bins.

7 Advise the patient that they are likely to experience urgency and urethral irritation when urinating but that this should settle in 24–48 hours.

8 Residual volumes should be measured by ultrasound after micturition and documented.

Suprapubic catheters

Suprapubic aspiration of urine and catheterisation was first described by Huze and Beeson in 1956 and advocated as a superior way to obtain a 'clean catch' of urine for bacterial culture. It is a relatively safe procedure but should only be performed by a competent healthcare professional.

Indications

- Urinary retention.
- Urine sampling in paediatrics.
- Phimosis.
- Chronic infection of urethra/periurethral glands.
- Urethral stricture.
- Urethral trauma.
- Post transurethral surgery.
- Resection of prostate.
- Neuropathic bladder.

Contraindications

- Known bladder tumour (can cause spread).
- Neobladder.
- Empty/indefinable bladder.
- Lower abdominal surgery/scarring.
- Pelvic irradiation.
- Unfamiliarity with procedure.
- Refusal of a competent patient.

Advantages over urethral catheterisation

- Reduced urethral stricture formation.
- Lower rates of infection – bacteriuria, pyelonephritis and urinary sepsis.
- Prevention of penile pressure necrosis.
- Reduced interference with sexual function.
- Possibly more acceptable to patients.

Step-by-step guide: insertion of suprapubic catheter

- **Give a full explanation to the patient in simple terms and ensure they consent to the procedure.**
- **Set up your trolley (Box 18.2).**
- **Prepare your trolley as a sterile field. Wear a plastic disposable apron and non-sterile gloves, and take alcohol hand rub with you.**

1 Give clear and simple explanations throughout. Lie the patient supine with the abdomen and pelvic area exposed. Children should be held in a supine frog-legged position (assistance for this will be needed). Wear sterile gloves and gown, considering also personal protective equipment such as eye protection.

2 Palpate 2 cm above the symphysis pubis in the midline for a full bladder. This should be confirmed by ultrasound and ideally the procedure done under ultrasound guidance, with the transducer covered with a sterile glove.

3 Clean the area using a circular motion and treat as a sterile field.

Box 18.2 **Additional equipment for the insertion of a suprapubic catheter**

In addition to the equipment listed in Box 18.1 you will need the following:
- ultrasound machine
- 22G needle
- local anaesthetic (e.g. 1% lidocaine)
- 10/20-mL sterile syringe
- scalpel
- cystostomy kit, these vary widely between various manufacturers, you should be familiar with the contents of the kit before you need to use it!
- catheter dressing.

4 Infiltrate the skin with local anaesthetic in the midline 2 cm superior from the pubic symphysis.

5 For aspiration, use a 22G needle (short length in children), attached to a 10/20-mL syringe. Advance the needle while aspirating until urine appears. In children the bladder is still an abdominal organ so the needle should be angled slightly towards the abdomen (cephalad). In adults the bladder is a pelvic organ so the needle should be angled slightly towards the pelvic floor (caudad). Once the sample is obtained, remove the needle and apply pressure with gauze before applying a sterile dressing to the site.

6 For suprapubic catheter insertion you will have a cystostomy kit as part of your equipment set up on your sterile tray. At the site of the aspiration, make a small incision with a scalpel.

7 Insert the trochar and cannula in the same direction as the aspiration needle until the bladder is entered and you aspirate urine.

8 Remove the trochar – urine should now gush out of the distended bladder. In some kits the cannula itself acts as the catheter which is sutured in place and connected to the drainage bag. In others, a Foley catheter is inserted through the cannula and the balloon inflated. The cannula then normally peels apart and can be removed.

9 Secure the catheter with a dressing.

Suprapubic catheterisation in a non-distended bladder can be performed after filling the bladder with saline via a flexible cystoscopy. Occasionally, particularly if there has been lower abdominal surgery, an open cystostomy under general anaesthetic is necessary.

Complications

These are rare but potentially serious.
- Infection: superficial of the skin and subcutaneous tissues, intra-abdominal or bladder.
- Peritoneal perforation with or without visceral injury. Can be potentially life-threatening if bowel is perforated and catheter left in place. A vesicocolic fistula may form.
- Haematuria: as with urethral catheterisation this is usually temporary and more commonly microscopic.
- Inability to aspirate urine: you will need to contact the urology team.

Table 18.1 Causes of oliguria and anuria.

Prerenal

Hypovolaemia

Hypotension

Renal artery stenosis (in combination with an ACE inhibitor)

Renal artery thrombosis

Hepatorenal syndrome

Renal

Acute tubular necrosis:
- ischaemic secondary to reduced renal perfusion
- toxins – e.g. myoglobin in rhabdomyolysis
- drugs (e.g. gentamicin)
- infection (e.g. malaria)

Vasculitis, for example:
- Wegener's
- Churg–Strauss
- Goodpasture's
- herpes simplex virus

Toxins:
- drugs – NSAIDs, diuretics
- calcium/oxalate

Postrenal

Ureteral obstruction

Bladder outlet obstruction

Renal calculi

Prostatic hypertrophy

Renal vein thrombosis

Why monitor urine output?

It is outside the scope of this book to discuss in full the monitoring of urine output. The production of urine is a reflection of fluid balance status of the body and how well the kidneys are functioning to excrete waste products and regulate fluid balance. A reduction in urine output is a signal that all is not physiologically normal in the body; this requires your attention.

Oliguria is a reduced urine output, defined as a urine output of less than 300 mL in 24 hours, or better, less than 0.5 mL/kg/hour. Anuria is the failure to produce any volume of urine and requires urgent attention. Causes of reduced urine output can be prerenal, renal and post-renal (Table 18.1).

Any patient with low urine output should be thoroughly assessed as to the likely cause. Oliguria for more than 2 hours is an emergency. If in doubt or the patient is not responding to initial treatment, get senior advice.

Handy hints/troubleshooting

- If the catheterisation is handed over to you out of hours, always take a brief history and examine the patient to ensure you are happy with the indications.
- Always check for allergies, especially latex.
- Take a drug history – if the patient is on anticoagulation haematuria secondary to catheterisation is more likely and may last longer.
- Take a chaperone who is the same sex as the patient, unless the patient has any objections.
- Some people use a double glove technique with one larger set of gloves over ones normal size as this saves time during the procedure.
- Consider the impact on sexual function, particularly in patients who may require long-term catheterisation – is suprapubic catheterisation more appropriate?

Further reading

Aguilera P, Choi T, Durham B. (2004) Ultrasound-guided cystostomy catheter placement in the emergency department. *Journal of Emergency Medicine* 26: 319–21.

Berne RM, Levy MN. (2000) *Principles of Physiology*, 3rd edn. Mosby Publishing, St Louis.

Blandy J. (1998) *Lecture Notes on Urology*. Blackwell Science, Oxford.

Brewster S, Cranston D, Noble J, Reynard J. (2001) *Urology: A Handbook for Medical Students*. Bios Scientific, Oxford.

Kumar P. Pati J. (2005) Suprapubic catheters: indications and complications. *Br J Hosp Med* 66: 466–8.

Mallet J, Doherty L. (2001) *The Royal Marsden NHS Trust: Manual of Clinical Nursing Procedures*, 5th edn. Blackwell Science, Oxford.

Roth D. (2006) *Suprapubic Aspiration*. www.emedicine.com/proc/topic82964.htm

CHAPTER 19

Monitoring: Central Line

Ronan O'Leary[1] and Andrew Quinn[2]

[1]*Yorkshire Deanery, York, UK*
[2]*Department of Anaesthesia, Bradford Royal Infirmary, Bradford, UK*

OVERVIEW

By the end of this chapter you should be able to:

- understand the use of central line monitoring in theatres and critical care settings
- understand how the central venous pulse waveform is directly related to the cardiac cycle
- use central venous pressure as a guide to fluid therapy to optimise cardiac function
- understand central venous oxygen saturations.

Introduction

Central venous catheters can be used for a number of physiological measurements and can aid the assessment and treatment of critically ill patients.

How does central venous pressure relate to cardiac filling?

Measurement of central venous pressure (CVP) is a frequently used tool in the management of critically ill and high-risk surgical patients. CVP is a reflection of the state of cardiac filling before ventricular contraction and a means of assessing the intravascular volume status of a patient. The CVP allows optimisation of cardiovascular function and can be used to guide fluid therapy during resuscitation.

Cardiac output (CO) is calculated in the following way:

$$\begin{matrix} \text{Cardiac output} = & \text{Heart rate} & \times & \text{Stroke volume} \\ \text{(CO) (L/min)} & \text{(HR)(beats/min)} & & \text{(SV) (L/stroke)} \end{matrix}$$

The determinants of CO are preload, afterload and contractility.
- **Preload** is the degree of filling of the heart during diastole.
- **Afterload** is the force the heart has to contract against to eject blood during systole; this is primarily due to systemic vascular resistance (SVR) or the 'tone' of the vascular system.
- **Contractility** is the ability of the heart muscle itself to alter the volume of blood ejected during each beat independent of the preload and afterload; essentially it is the inotropic state of the heart.

Critically ill patients will often have a poor CO, but this can be optimised in a number of ways.
- **Preload** can be altered by varying the volume of fluid filling of the heart during diastole.
- **Afterload** can be manipulated by using **vasodilators** and **vasoconstrictors**.
- **Contractility** can be increased by the use of **inotropes** which act to increase the calcium concentration within the myocyte and increase the force of contraction.

The CVP gives us an estimation of preload. The tip of the catheter should lie in a central vein, i.e. a large, intrathoracic vein close to the heart which lacks valves. The CVP therefore gives an estimate of right atrial pressure, since there is a continuous column of blood between its tip and the right atrium.

If preload is increased, the stroke volume will increase. This relationship is described by the Frank–Starling law. This states that the force of contraction is related to the initial muscle fibre length. If the muscle fibres of the heart are stretched by increasing the preload, the force of contraction exerted by these muscle fibres will increase. Therefore, when the heart rate is constant and afterload is unaltered, CO is directly proportional to preload. This applies until excessive end-diastolic volumes are reached when CO no longer increases and eventually decreases: the failing heart (Figure 19.1).

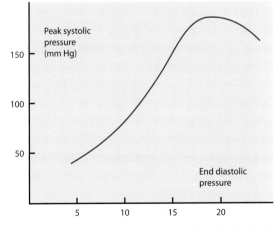

Figure 19.1 Frank–Starling curve: the curve shows that the relationship between preload and stroke volume is linear until a plateau is reached where the heart is working at peak efficiency – further increases in preload do not improve CO. CVP monitoring guides fluid therapy to allow the plateau portion of the Starling curve to be reached.

ABC of Practical Procedures. Edited by T. Nutbeam and R. Daniels. © 2010 Blackwell Publishing, ISBN: 978-1-4051-8595-0.

Improving the CO of critically ill patients improves oxygen delivery to the tissues and organs. In some studies, particularly in septic shock, this has been shown to decrease morbidity and mortality.

Measurement of central venous pressure

The CVP is the pressure within the superior vena cava (SVC) just above the right atrium. It is impossible without imaging to determine the precise position of the SVC–atrial boundary and the position of the end of the central venous tip in each patient, and then to relate this to the body surface. Therefore it is standard practice to take all measurements at the same level in all patients. In the supine patient the pressure is measured from the fourth intercostal space in the mid-axillary line which is taken to be the level of the right atrium.

The normal range of CVP is 3–10 cmH$_2$O. Previously, this pressure was measured by attaching the central line to a water-filled manometer but this has been superseded by electronic pressure transducers that are able to display the CVP waveform in real-time.

Pressure transducers

Pressure transducers consist of a length of tubing with a transducer situated at the midpoint between the patient and a bag of fluid under pressure (Figure 19.2). At the patient end, the giving set is attached to the central venous catheter and the other end is attached to a bag of pressurised saline. Saline flows down the tubing, limited by a flow regulator within the transducer that allows a flow of 3 mL per hour. This prevents the formation of blood clots within the catheter.

In order to display the CVP waveform on a monitor, the pressure wave has to be converted into an electrical signal. A transducer converts one form of energy into another. In this case, mechanical energy in the form of the central venous pressure is converted to electrical energy which is displayed as a waveform on the monitor.

The measuring system must be zeroed to atmospheric pressure before use. The transducer is usually placed at the level of the right atrium, as described above. If the patient's position is altered by raising or lowering the bed or operating table, the transducer must be moved with it to the new level of the mid-axillary line (repeating the zero each time is unnecessary).

CVP waveform

The central venous pulsation is a complex waveform which differs in many respects from the arterial pulsation. It is described as having three positive deflections ('a', 'c' and 'v') and two negative deflections ('x' and 'y'). Figure 19.3 explains what causes these deflections and how they are related to the ECG.

The CVP waveform displays abnormal morphology during various pathological states (Box 19.1). The point on the CVP waveform which most accurately reflects cardiac preload is just before the 'c' wave. This is the point just before the tricuspid valve closes and before ventricular systole begins. The pressure at this point

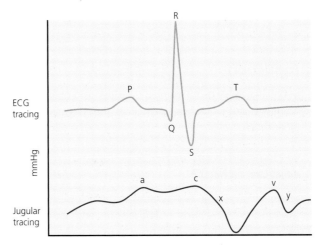

Figure 19.3 **+a wave**: due to right atrial contraction and is not seen in patients with atrial fibrillation. It correlates with the P wave on an ECG.
+c wave: a result of closure and bulging of the tricuspid valve during isovolumetric contraction of the right ventricle. It correlates with the end of the QRS segment on an ECG.
−x descent: due to atrial relaxation and descent of the tricuspid annulus during ventricular contraction. It occurs before the T wave on an ECG.
+v wave: result of continuing filling of the right atrium against the closed tricuspid valve. It occurs as the T wave is ending on an ECG.
−y descent: due to the tricuspid valve opening and rapid ventricular filling. It occurs before the P wave on an ECG.

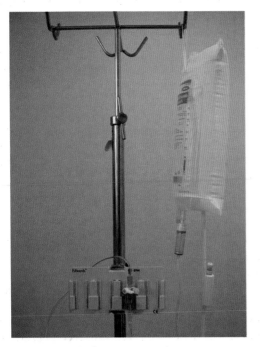

Figure 19.2 A photograph of a pressure transducer set up.

Box 19.1 **Abnormal CVP waveforms**

- Cannon waves   AV dissociation/junctional rhythm/VT/pacing
- Large 'a' waves   Tricuspid stenosis/pulmonary stenosis/ pulmonary hypertension/right ventricular failure/right atrial myxoma
- Large 'v' waves   Tricuspid incompetence
- Rapid 'x' descent   Cardiac tamponade/constrictive pericarditis
- Rapid 'y' descent   Constrictive pericarditis

Box 19.2 Causes of high and low CVPs

Raised CVP >15 cm H$_2$O
- Hypervolaemia
- Heart failure
- Right ventricular infarction
- Cor pulmonale/right ventricular failure
- Constrictive pericarditis/restrictive cardiomyopathy
- Pulmonary embolus
- SVC obstruction
- Intermittent positive pressure ventilation
- Tricuspid incompetence

Lowered CVP <3 cm H$_2$O
- Acute hypovolaemia e.g. haemorrhage
- High-output cardiac failure e.g. sepsis, thyrotoxicosis
- Decreased sympathetic tone e.g. anaphylaxis, spinal anaesthesia, spinal shock
- Drugs, e.g. vasodilators (GTN, sodium nitroprusside)

Box 19.3 Factors affecting CVP

Central venous blood volume
- Venous return/cardiac output
- Total blood volume
- Regional vascular tone

Compliance of central compartment
- Vascular tone
- Right ventricular compliance
  - Myocardial disease
  - Pericardial disease
  - Tamponade

Tricuspid valve disease
- Stenosis
- Regurgitation

Cardiac rhythm
- Junctional rhythm
- AF
- A–V dissociation

Reference level of transducer
- Positioning of patient

Intrathoracic pressure
- Respiration
- Intermittent positive pressure ventilation (IPPV)
- Positive end-expiratory pressure (PEEP)
- Tension pneumothorax

correlates with right ventricular end-diastolic pressure, i.e. a measure of preload.

Factors affecting central venous pressure

There are various factors that affect the measurement of CVP. These include the intravascular volume and venous return as well as the vascular tone of the venous system. Any increase in vascular tone will result in a pressure rise within the venous capacitance system and lead to a rise in CVP.

The CVP is subject to swings because of the transmission of pressure from the lungs to the SVC during respiration. During the inspiratory phase the pressure within the thoracic cavity decreases to facilitate gas flow into the lungs and this in turn causes a drop in CVP. These changes may frequently be reversed in critically ill patients ventilated on intensive care because of the positive pressure used during the inspiratory phase of mechanical ventilation. These patients may have positive end-expiratory pressure (PEEP) applied as part of their respiratory support which also increases the measured CVP.

Additionally, abnormalities of the tricuspid valve, cardiac rhythm and myocardial pathology may lead to erroneous CVP measurement and waveforms (Box 19.2).

Interpretation of the CVP

When interpreting the CVP, the actual value is less important than the trend that emerges with response to therapy. There are a variety of patient factors that contribute to variations in CVP, for example the stiffness of the ventricular wall, the position of the catheter, the position of the patient, the intrapulmonary pressures, etc. In practice, the measured CVP value is often not used as a direct measure of preload but as a guide to the likelihood of a patient responding to fluid therapy.

A low CVP can be indicative of acute hypovolaemic states, high-output cardiac failure states, decreased sympathetic tone or the use of vasodilatory drugs. A raised CVP can be as a result of fluid therapy (see below) or can have various pathological causes (see Box 19.3).

When fluid is administered it is important to note the trend of the change in the CVP and also to see if any increase in the CVP is sustained over time.

Transient rise in CVP with fluid bolus—Indicates that the right ventricle is operating on the ascending part of the Starling curve and therefore more fluid will be needed to optimise cardiac preload.

Sustained rise in CVP with fluid bolus—The plateau part of the Starling curve has been reached. If a patient's cardiac function is still inadequate after a sustained increase in the CVP then inotropes may be needed to improve myocardial contractility further.

Marked rise in CVP with clinical deterioration—The heart is beginning to fail due to excessive preload and overstretching of the muscle fibres. Cardiac output is decreasing and is likely to require support with inotropes and possibly vasodilators and diuretics.

Mixed venous oxygen saturation

Oxygen delivery to the tissues is dependent on a combination of the following: cardiac output, the amount of oxygen in the blood and haemoglobin concentration.

Critical illness can cause a decrease in oxygen delivery due to a reduction in each of these factors. When oxygen delivery is decreased so that it does not meet demand, tissues compensate by increasing their percentage oxygen extraction from each mL of blood passing through the tissue and as a consequence the venous

Box 19.4 **Interpretation of mixed venous oxygen saturation**

Decreased mixed venous oxygen saturation (<65%)
- Low cardiac output states (e.g. hypovoalemia, myocardial infarction, heart failure)
- Hypoxia, respiratory distress syndromes
- Increased oxygen consumption (e.g. fever, exercise, thyrotoxicosis)
- Low Hb (e.g. bleeding, haemolysis)

Increased mixed venous oxygen saturation (>80%)
- High cardiac output (e.g. sepsis, burns, inotrope excess, hepatitis, pancreatitis and left-to-right shunts)
- Low oxygen consumption (e.g. cyanide toxicity, carbon monoxide poisoning, sepsis and hypothermia)

Box 19.5 **Hagen–Poiseuille equation**

The rate of flow of fluid through a catheter is described by the Hagen–Poiseuille equation. This states that the flow is directly proportional to the radius of the catheter to its fourth power and the pressure gradient along the infusion tubing. Flow is also inversely proportional to the length of the catheter and the viscosity of the fluid being infused.

$$Flow = \frac{\Delta P \pi r^4}{8 \eta l}$$

P = pressure difference along the catheter
r = radius of catheter
l = length of catheter
η = viscosity of liquid
π = constant

oxygen saturation of mixed venous blood will fall from the normal range of 68–77%.

Blood from a central venous catheter taken with an arterial blood gas syringe can be used to estimate mixed venous saturations. (The saturation measured in this way is slightly higher than true mixed venous blood as it does not include the deoxygenated blood from the cardiac and pulmonary circulations; Box 19.4.)

Fluid resuscitation

Unless peripheral venous access is problematic, central venous catheters should not routinely be used for fluid resuscitation especially where the patient is shocked due to haemorrhage. The flow of fluid through a central line is too slow to allow rapid administration of fluids or blood products (Box 19.5).

Clinical examples of data interpretation

Example 1: The septic, hypotensive patient

A 25-year-old man was admitted with an area of spreading cellulitis to his leg which developed into necrotising fasciitis.

On assessment by the intensive care team his observations were: heart rate 140 bpm, blood pressure 75/45 mmHg and CVP 2 cmH_2O. On examination he appeared flushed and was noted to have a bounding pulse. A diagnosis of sepsis causing hypotension and vasodilatation was made. The hypotension was due to a decrease in systemic vascular resistance (SVR) due to septic mediators.

He was given several fluid boluses (250–500 mL of crystalloid) which provided only a transient increase in CVP and BP. His treatment would require further fluid boluses and a vasoconstrictor infusion via the central line to increase his SVR and perfusion pressure to his organs.

Example 2: The trauma patient

A 40-year-old woman was admitted following a road traffic accident. Her injuries included a fractured femur and bilateral chest trauma. The results of the primary survey were that her airway was safe, she had a right-sided pneumothorax which was decompressed using an intercostal drain, and she was hypotensive (BP 86/55 mmHg) and tachycardic (HR 130).

After several fluid boluses she remained hypotensive but stable. It was decided to insert a central venous catheter to aid further fluid resuscitation. The initial CVP reading was 20 mmHg and it was then noted that her neck veins were distended whilst at the same time she started to display increasing respiratory distress.

Further examination revealed absent breath sounds on the left and a hyperresonant chest. A left tension pneumothorax was successfully decompressed which immediately resulted in a reduction of CVP and an increase in blood pressure.

Further reading

Pinsky MR, Payen D. (2005) *Update in Intensive Care and Emergency Medicine 42: Functional Haemodynamic Monitoring.* Springer Verlag, Berlin, Heidleberg.

Rivers E, Nguyen B, Havstad S, Ressler J, Mussin A, Knoblich B. (2001) Early goal-directed therapy in the treatment of sepsis and septic shock. *N Engl J Med* 345: 1371–7.

CHAPTER 20

Monitoring: Arterial Line

Rob Moss

Mersey Rotation, Liverpool, UK

OVERVIEW

By the end of this chapter you should be able to:

- understand the indications and contraindications for insertion of an arterial line
- understand the anatomy of the relevant sites of insertion
- describe the two commonly used types of arterial cannulae
- describe the procedure of inserting an arterial line
- interpret an arterial waveform.

Introduction

Arterial lines are routinely used in the operating theatre and intensive care settings in the monitoring of critically ill patients. They allow beat-to-beat display of heart rate and blood pressure, as well as sampling of arterial blood for analysis without the need for repeated arterial puncture.

Indications

Theatre

- Major surgical cases.
- Cardiovascular instability.
- Moderate or severe ischaemic heart disease.
- Cerebrovascular disease.
- Acid–base disturbances (particularly emergencies).
- Likely need for inotropic (or vasopressor) support.
- Hypotensive anaesthesia.
- Failure of non-invasive blood pressure measurement.

Intensive care

- Inotropic (or vasopressor) support.
- Frequent arterial blood gas sampling.
- Monitoring of waveform for cardiac output and end-diastolic volume estimation.

Contraindications

The risks associated with arterial cannulation must be balanced with the benefits that can be gained. The patient's coagulation status should be considered as haemorrhage may be difficult to control and a haematoma can also lead to distal ischaemia. Arterial cannulation should be avoided:

- in limbs where the collateral circulation has been demonstrated to be poor
- where there is active infection or ischaemia
- where there is a surgical shunt, such as for renal dialysis.

Anatomy and sites

A number of superficial arteries are suitable for catheterisation with an arterial cannula. The most commonly used site is the radial artery at the wrist, ideally of the non-dominant hand. Other sites include brachial, axillary, ulnar, dorsalis pedis and femoral arteries. The radial artery is preferred due to its ease of location in its superficial position at the distal end of the radius between the tendons of the brachioradialis and flexor carpi radialis. The cannula site can also be readily inspected. Importantly the tissues supplied by the radial artery have a collateral circulation, via the ulnar artery, which helps to minimise the risk of ischaemic damage should the radial artery thrombose following cannulation.

The collateral supply of the ulnar artery can be demonstrated using the modified Allen test (see Box 20.1 and Figure 20.1) or by using a Doppler probe, before cannulation of the radial artery. However, the Allen test has been demonstrated to have a poor sensitivity and specificity for ischaemic complications.

Equipment

The monitoring system consists of the arterial cannula, connected to a pressurised column of fluid with an inbuilt pressure transducer, and a monitor for display of the waveform.

Box 20.1 **Modified Allen's test**

Occlude the patient's radial and ulnar arteries simultaneously by direct pressure whilst exanguinating the hand through elevation and by asking the patient to make a fist. In an unconscious patient the hand can be squeezed so it blanches. With the hand open, release the pressure on the ulnar artery and observe the return in colour, which should occur within 6 seconds.

ABC of Practical Procedures. Edited by T. Nutbeam and R. Daniels. © 2010
Blackwell Publishing, ISBN: 978-1-4051-8595-0.

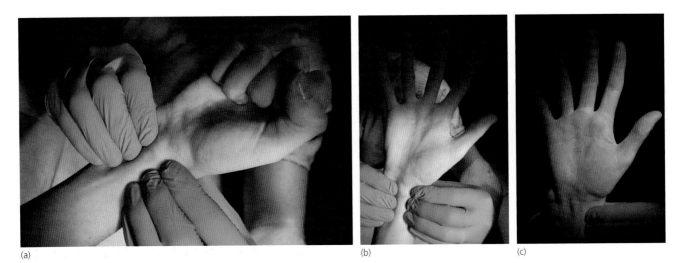

(a)   (b)   (c)

Figure 20.1 Allen's test. (a) The patient's hand is elevated and pressure applied to both the radial and ulnar arteries. (b) The patient's hand will blanch white. (c) On release of pressure over the ulnar artery the hand should reperfuse and lose its white colouration.

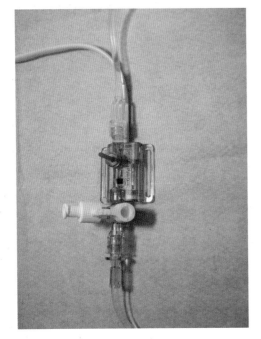

Figure 20.2 An arterial transducer.

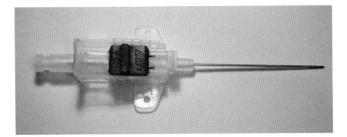

Figure 20.3 A FloSwitch™ type arterial cannula.

The fluid is pressurised to 300 mmHg, and the giving set incorporates a continuous flush system at 4 mL/h to help prevent clot formation and resultant waveform dampening. There is also a manual flush for clearing blood from the system after sampling.

A number of types of Teflon-coated arterial cannulae are available that differ in their mechanism of insertion. Most arterial cannulae differ from venous in that the ends of the cannulae are square rather than tapered. In younger patients particularly, it may be helpful to make a small stab incision into the skin to avoid the cannula tip catching.

The most commonly used types of cannulae in the UK are:
- **FloSwitch™** (Becton-Dickinson UK) which looks similar to a venous cannula but with a switch for occluding flow, and is inserted in a manner similar to venous cannulation (Figure 20.3)
- **Leader cath™** (Vygon UK) which is a longer cannula, up to 10 cm, that is inserted using the Seldinger cannula over wire technique (Figure 20.4).

The type of cannula used and method of insertion is often down to personal preference. Both cannulae have a maximum size of 20G in order to minimise the risk of thrombosis and arterial occlusion.

The arterial pulsations are transmitted along the column of fluid to the transducer, which converts the pressure changes into an electrical signal displayed as the arterial waveform (Figure 20.2).

The tubing containing the column of fluid is of a specific compliance in order to produce the optimum waveform. There is a three-way tap included to allow for arterial blood sampling without disconnection. Either heparinised or normal saline can be used as the system fluid. More centres are now discarding heparinised solutions since there is little evidence of benefit.

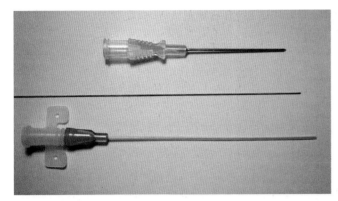

Figure 20.4 A Seldinger type arterial cannula (Leader cath™).

Box 20.2 **Equipment for insertion of arterial cannula**

Prepare using aseptic no-touch technique wearing non-sterile gloves and apron.
- Sterile drapes
- Sterile gloves
- Gauze
- Skin antiseptic solution
- Arterial cannula
- Lidocaine 1%
- 25G needle for lidocaine infiltration
- 5-mL syringe
- Saline flush
- Suture
- Dressing
- Pressurised transducer system

Step-by-step guide: insertion of arterial cannula

A suitable site should be chosen by examining the patient and assessing for any contraindications.

- **Give a full explanation to the patient in simple terms and ensure they consent to the procedure (if able).**
- **Set up your trolley (Box 20.2 and Figure 20.5).**
- **Ensure the pressurised monitoring system is set up.**
- **Prepare your trolley as a sterile field. Wear a plastic disposable apron and non-sterile gloves, and take alcohol hand rub with you.**

Insertion at the radial artery (the most commonly used site) is described first using the FloSwitch™ cannula.

1 After setting up the trolley, discard gloves and apron used, rewash hands and don a new pair of non-sterile gloves and apron.
2 Before putting on sterile gloves, position the patient with the wrist dorsiflexed (Figure 20.6a). This can be achieved using a rolled towel or bag of intravenous fluid placed under the forearm with the hand taped, hyperextended, to the bed.

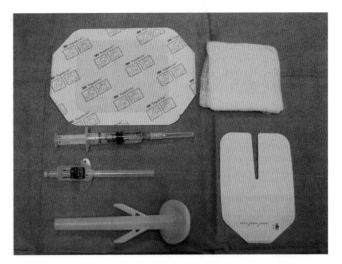

Figure 20.5 Equipment for insertion of arterial cannula.

3 Don sterile gloves. Clean the wrist with a skin antiseptic (2% chlorhexidine in 70% isopropyl alcohol is recommended) and drape the area (Figure 20.6b). A sterile technique should be maintained throughout insertion and securing the cannula.
4 Palpate the radial artery and infiltrate local anaesthetic (0.5–1 mL 1% lidocaine) subcutaneously (Figure 20.6c,d).
5 Whilst palpating the artery with the non-dominant hand hold the arterial cannula like a pencil with the bevel facing up the arm. Puncture the skin at an angle of 30–40° (Figure 20.6e).
6 Advance the needle until a flashback of blood is seen in the hub of the needle (Figure 20.6f).
7 The cannula can then be advanced off the needle up the lumen of the artery (Figure 20.6g).

Alternatively, a transfixing technique can be used whereby the needle and cannula pass through both walls of the artery. This is described below and in Figure 20.7, omitting step **7** above.

7 Continue to advance the needle deeper through the arterial lumen and a further few millimetres out of the other side of the artery so the artery is now transfixed by the cannula.
8 Keeping the cannula in position, withdraw the needle until the tip of the needle can be seen at the level of the skin.
9 Flatten the angle of the cannula down to 10–20° to the skin and slowly withdraw the cannula. As the tip of the cannula is pulled back into the lumen of the artery a flash of blood will be seen in the cannula lumen indicating that the tip of the cannula is in the arterial lumen.
10 The cannula can then be gently advanced up the lumen of the artery.
11 Remove the needle, disposing of it safely, closing the FloSwitch™ to prevent blood loss.

For cannulation using the Seldinger technique for a Leader cath™ the preparation is the same up to step **3**, then:
4 Whilst palpating the artery with the non-dominant hand puncture the skin, at an angle of 30–40°, with the supplied 20G needle.

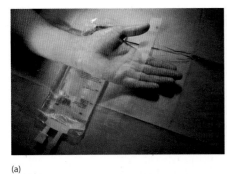
(a)

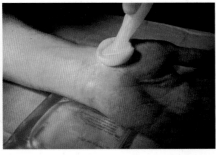
(b)

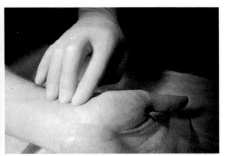
(c)

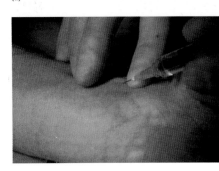
(d)

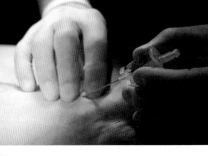
(e)

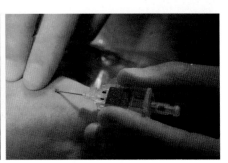
(f)

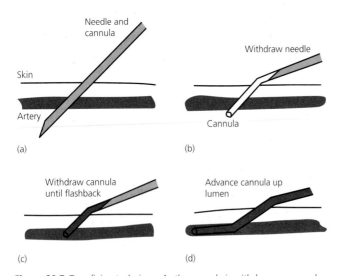
(g)

(h)

Figure 20.6 Step-by-step guide: insertion of arterial cannula. (a) The patient positioned with the wrist dorsiflexed. (b) Sterilising the wrist with 2% chlorhexidine in 70% isopropyl alcohol solution. (c) Palpating the radial artery to identify the point of maximal pulsation. (d) Infiltrating local anaesthetic (0.5–1 mL 1% lidocaine) subcutaneously. (e) Puncturing the skin at an angle of 30–40°. (f) Advancing the needle until a flashback of blood is seen in the hub of the needle. (g) Advancing the cannula off the needle up the lumen of the artery. (h) Dressed cannula with sterile dressing.

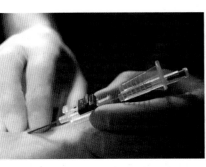

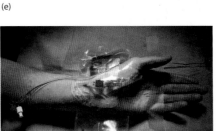

(a)

(b)

(c)

(d)

Figure 20.7 Transfixing technique. As the cannula is withdrawn a secondary flashback is seen.

5 Advance the needle until the artery is punctured giving a free pulsating flow of blood.

6 Pass the guidewire through the needle and up the artery so that majority of the guidewire is in the artery lumen (Figure 20.8a).

7 Withdraw the needle completely whilst maintaining the position of the guidewire in the artery. Place the cannula over the guidewire whilst holding the guidewire at the level of the skin and advance the cannula towards your fingers (Figure 20.8b). Feed the wire back through the cannula until it protrudes from the hub of the cannula and then, taking care to maintain a hold on the guidewire, advance the cannula over the guidewire into the lumen of the artery. A rotational motion helps advance the cannula.

8 Remove the guidewire and cap the end of the cannula to prevent blood loss (Figure 20.8c).

The cannula can then be secured, with sutures if required, and covered with a semipermeable sterile dressing that allows visual inspection (Figure 20.6h).

The pressurised fluid system is then connected to the cannula, not forgetting to open the FloSwitch™, allowing the cannula to be flushed.

The system must then be zeroed to give an accurate reading. The pressure transducer is put at the same level as the patient's heart, and the three-way tap is closed off towards the patient and opened towards atmospheric air allowing the system to be zeroed.

The procedure including aseptic precautions and any complications should be documented.

Complications

The most common complication of arterial catheterisation is thrombosis which occurs in up to 30% of cases. The risk of thrombosis increases with the diameter of the cannula and the duration it remains in place. Haematoma formation occurs both after insertion and after removal and can be reduced through minimising movement of the catheter and by applying adequate pressure after removal. As the risk of infection at the site of puncture increases with the duration of placement, cannulae should not be left in place longer than absolutely necessary.

Arterial waveform

Information other than simply the systolic and diastolic blood pressures and heart rate can be gained from inspecting the shape of the arterial waveform (Figure 20.9). The slope of the upstroke of the waveform reflects the contractility of the myocardium, with a poorly contracting heart having a less steep slope. Cardiac output can be estimated by multiplying the area underneath the waveform before the dichrotic notch (the stroke volume) by the heart rate. In hypovolaemic patients the dichrotic notch is lowered; the slope of the waveform after the dichrotic notch reflects the degree of vasoconstriction of the patient, with a gentle sloping waveform seen in patients who are vasoconstricted. The mean arterial blood pressure – the average pressure over the length of the cardiac cycle – is calculated by integrating the pressure wave.

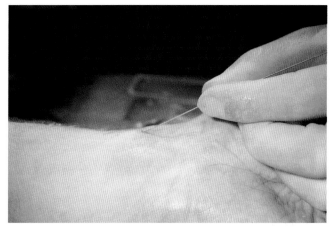

(a)

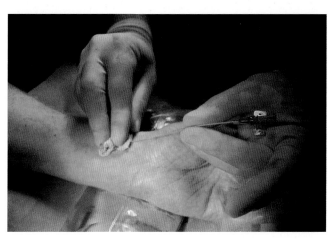

(b)

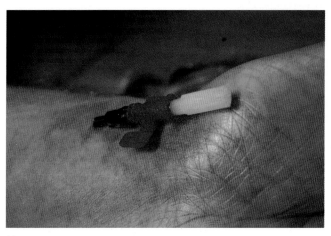

(c)

Figure 20.8 Seldinger technique. (a) A Seldinger wire in the artery is used as a guide for the insertion of the cannula. (b) The cannula is inserted over the wire. (c) The Seldinger type cannula in final position (with bung inserted).

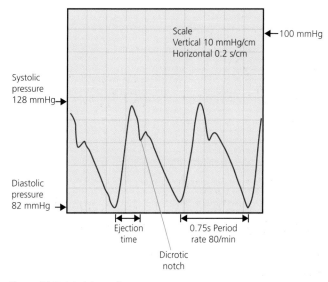

Figure 20.9 Arterial waveform.

Handy hints/troubleshooting

- Have a few cannulae of different types to hand, as frequent attempts may be needed in difficult cases.
- Have plenty of gauze ready to catch blood loss.
- Palpate lightly so as to not obliterate flow.
- If the cannula, or guidewire, will not advance, aspirate with a 5-mL syringe and withdraw slowly until pulsatile flow is found before attempting to advance the cannula again.
- If a FloSwitch™ cannula is sited in the vessel but fails to advance fully, conversion to a Seldinger technique by passing the guidewire through the device may help.
- The artery may go into spasm; if so, change site or wait until the pulse returns.
- Limit your number of attempts to minimise damage to the vessel.
- Don't forget to apply pressure to puncture sites for at least 3 minutes after failed attempts and removal.

Further reading

Davis PD, Kenny GNC. (2003) *Basic Physics and Measurement in Anaesthesia.* Butterworth Heinmann.

Mandel M, Dauchot P. (1977) Radial artery cannulation in 1000 patients: precautions and complications. *J Hand Surgery* 12s: 482–5.

Martin C, Saux P, Papazian L, Gouin F. (2001) Long-term arterial cannulation in ICU patients using the radial artery or dorsalis pedis artery. *Chest* 119(3): 901–6.

Steele A. (1999) Arterial blood gases and acid–base balance: Allen's test is not routinely used before radial artery puncture. *BMJ* 318(7185): 734.

Tuncali BE, Kuvaki B, Tuncali B, Capar E. (2005) A comparison of the efficacy of heparinized and nonheparinized solutions for maintenance of perioperative radial arterial catheter patency and subsequent occlusion. *Anesth Analg* 100(4): 1117–21.

CHAPTER 21

Specials: Suturing and Joint Aspiration

Simon Laing[1] and Chris Hetherington[2]

[1]*City Hospital, Birmingham, UK*
[2]*Worcestershire Acute Hospitals NHS Trust, Alexandra Hospital, Redditch, UK*

OVERVIEW

By the end of this chapter you should be able to:
- identify which wounds to suture
- describe and identify the equipment needed
- describe how to suture
- know which joints to aspirate
- describe how to aspirate a joint.

Suturing

Wounds are caused by several mechanisms. A focused history and examination will assess:
- indications for, and contraindications to closure in the emergency department
- the most appropriate method of wound closure.

Wound closure

- Primary closure: prompt surgical closure (i.e. immediate suturing of wound).
- Delayed primary closure: closure 3–5 days post injury.
- Secondary closure: healing by secondary intention i.e. via formation of granulation tissue.

   Primary closure approximates wounds as accurately as possible. It aims for the best possible cosmetic result and to assist the healing process.

Indications (suitable wounds)

- Wounds created by sharp metal/knife/glass.
- Wounds overlying cosmetically unimportant areas (e.g. scalp laceration).
- Healthy wound edges (good blood supply).
- Base of the wound is visible.
- No neurovascular deficit.
- No or minimal tissue loss.

Contraindications (unsuitable wounds)

- Associated tendinous or bony injury.
- Presence of foreign material.
- Infected/dirty wound.
- Inability to adequately clean/explore wound with facilities/local anaesthetic alone.
- Irregular edges which are difficult to approximate accurately.
- Crush injuries.
- Wounds more than 12 hours since injury.

Other options to suturing

Steristrips (Figure 21.1)
- Wounds with well approximated edges which will oppose with minimal tension (e.g. pretibial skinflap).
- Unsuitable on hairy areas.
- Need to be kept dry for 7 days.

Skin tissue adhesive/glue (e.g. histoacryl)

- Applied only to the upper epidermis.
- Often used in conjunction with steristrips.

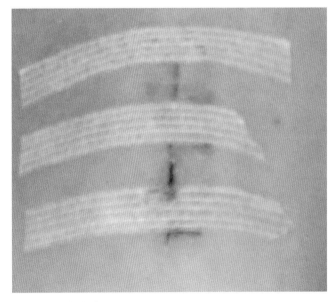

Figure 21.1 Steristrips.

ABC of Practical Procedures. Edited by T. Nutbeam and R. Daniels. © 2010
Blackwell Publishing, ISBN: 978-1-4051-8595-0.

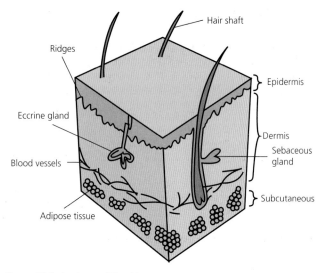

Figure 21.2 Anatomy of the skin.

- Useful in children (eliminating the need to inject local anaesthetic).
- Needs to be kept dry for 7 days.

Metal clips

These are infrequently used outside of the operating theatre.

Anatomy of the skin

The skin is composed of three histologically distinct layers (Figure 21.2).

Epidermis—A stratified squamous epithelium with epidermal ridges.

Dermis—The dermis is subdivided into papillary and reticular layers. The papillary layer houses small blood vessels, lymphatics and nerve cells sets within fine collagen and elastic fibres. It also contains invaginations of epithelium. The reticular layer consists of a vascular plexus, lymph and nerve cells embedded in thicker elastic fibres and a dense collagen network; it is within this layer that sweat glands and hair follicles originate.

Subcutaneous layer/hypodermis—This consists predominantly of adipose tissue.

Suture types

Absorbable sutures, such as vicryl and monocryl, can be used to close deep layers of dermis and will not require removal.

Non-absorbable sutures, such as nylon and prolene, are frequently used to close the epidermis and require subsequent removal. Choose the thickness of the suture material depending on the site being sutured. As a rough guide:

- lips and mouth 6/0
- facial 5/0 or 6/0
- hands and limbs 4/0
- scalp 2/0 or 3/0
- other sites 2/0 or 3/0.

Box 21.1 **Equipment for suturing**

Many hospitals have a suture pack which contains all the equipment you need – you should familiarise yourself with the packs available at your hospital.
As a minimum you require:
- topical antiseptic (e.g. 2% chlorhexidine in 70% alcohol)
- wound cleaning agent (normal saline will usually suffice)
- local anaesthetic (e.g. 1% lidocaine)
- sterile drapes
- needle holder, toothed forceps, scissors, gauze, gallipot
- sutures.

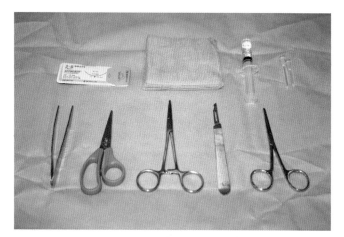

Figure 21.3 Equipment required to suture a wound.

Step-by-step guide: suturing

- **Give a full explanation to the patient in simple terms and ensure they consent to the procedure.**
- **Set up your trolley (Box 21.1 and Figure 21.3).**
- **Prepare your trolley as a sterile field. Wear a plastic disposable apron and sterile gloves, and take alcohol hand rub with you**

Preparation

1. Position the patient comfortably, with the wound on a secure surface if possible.
2. Ensure the field is adequately lit, adopt universal precautions, administer local anaesthesia and set a sterile field (as mentioned in previous chapters) (Figure 21.4).
3. Adequately clean the skin with an appropriate antiseptic solution (e.g. 2% chlorhexidine in 70% alcohol), irrigate the wound (with sterile saline) to remove foreign material and debride as appropriate.
4. Hold the needle holder with your dominant hand.
5. The needle holder should be held in a similar manner to scissors: thumb through one ring, ring finger through the other, with the index and middle fingers against the shaft of the holder for support to provide stability.

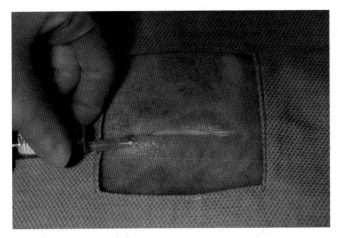

Figure 21.4 Administering local anaesthetic.

Your toothed forceps are held with your non-dominant hand, in between thumb and index finger, as a pincer grip, as you would a pen.

6 Pick up the needle with the forceps and mount it on the needle holder, approximately two-thirds of the way along its length from its tip, holding it at 90° to the needle holder.

NB suturing should be performed without handling the sharp with your hands, thus reducing the risk of injury – 'no-touch technique'.

7 If the wound is deep, absorbable sutures can be placed through the fascia before closing skin to eliminate potential spaces. This can be done with the same suture technique as described below.

8 The placement of the first suture is the most important; as a rule it should be at the middle of the wound, ensuring accurate alignment.

9 With a simple straight wound, it is easiest to position yourself so that it runs horizontally to your eye line.

Suturing

1 With the forceps, pick up the distal wound edge and evert it, holding it slightly raised.

2 With your dominant hand pronated, pierce the skin a reasonable distance from the wound edge; this should be equal to the depth of the bite required (approximately 2–10 mm, depending on the site, size and depth of wound and delicacy of suture material) and enter the skin at 90° (Figure 21.5a).

3 Supinate your dominant hand forming an arc; the needle should appear in the centre of the wound at an equal depth to the distance in step **2** (Figure 21.5b).

4 Ensuring the majority of the needle is visible in the base of the wound, release the needle from the needle holder.

5 Remount the needle on your needle holder.

6 Only once the needle is remounted may you release the distal skin edge from your forceps.

7 Pick up the proximal skin edge with your forceps and evert it. (Ideally the path taken by the suture through the proximal wound edge should mirror that of the path you have just taken through the distal wound edge.)

8 Insert the needle into the open surface of the wound at a similar distance from the skin edge to before.

9 Supinate your dominant hand, taking a path through the proximal skin edge with the needle emerging an equal distance from the wound edge as taken in step **2** (Figure 21.5b). NB avoid trapping excessive subcuticular tissue within the suture, as this will prevent accurate apposition of wound edges and will ultimately necrose, increasing infection risk.

10 Without moving the forceps, release the needle holder, then remount the needle on the side that has emerged from the wound.

11 Pull the majority of the suture through the wound, leaving a length of suture about 3–5 cm on the distal side of the wound edge (Figure 21.5c).

Now the suture must be tied to secure it as described below.

Knot tying: knot over forceps method

1 Position the needle holder parallel to the wound, raised a few centimetres above it.

2 With the longer length of suture (needle end) on the proximal side of the wound, wind this twice **clockwise** around the needle holder (do this holding the suture and not the needle) (Figure 21.5d).

3 Grasp the short end of the suture with the needle holder, pulling it through the two loops just created, so that the short end now lies on the proximal side of the wound and the long length on the distal side (i.e. cross hands). This 'tie' or 'throw' should lie flush against the skin (Figure 21.5e,f).

4 The knot should be pulled so that the wound edges just approximate.

Now secure the knot as follows.

5 Wind the long length of suture once **anticlockwise** around the needle holder. Again grasp the short end of the thread with the needle holder, pulling it through the single loop just created (again crossing hands). This throw should also lie flat, thus creating a 'squared' knot. This resembles a reef knot. If it resembles a slipknot, it has been done incorrectly (Figure 21.5g,h).

6 Finally wind the suture once **clockwise** around the needle holder pulling the short end through the loop to lock the knot.

7 Cut the two ends of thread 5 mm away from the knot.

Repeat your interrupted suturing until the wound is adequately opposed. Ensure that the wound edges are opposed correctly, everted and not overlapping. Failure to do so will prevent adequate healing. To ensure the knots do not scar, ensure removal at appropriate time periods. For example:

- lip   3 days
- face   3 days
- hands   10 days
- scalp   5 days
- other   7–10 days.

Complications
Early
- Wound malalignment.
- Suture displacement.

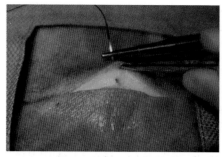

(a)

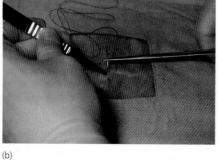

(b)

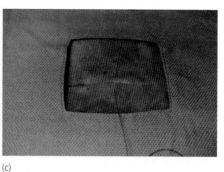

(c)

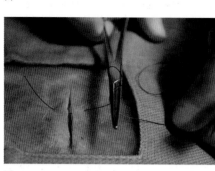

(d)

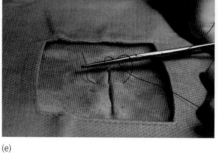

(e)

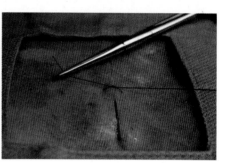

(f)

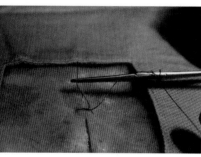

(g)

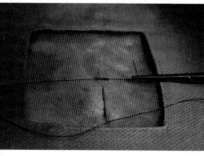

(h)

Figure 21.5 Step-by-step guide: suturing. (a) Initial insertion of needle (with eversion of distal wound edge). (b) Insertion of needle through proximal wound edge. (c) Position of suture – length of 3–5 cm on distal edge. (d) Two clockwise turns of suture over needle holder. (e) Grasping the short end of suture with needle holder. (f) Forming the first knot. (g) Securing knot with anticlockwise turn of suture over needle holder. (h) Securing the knot.

- Bleeding/haematoma formation.
- Inversion/overlapping of wound edges.
- 'Dog-earing' – this is where there is a unilateral excess of wound edge left over, caused by poorly placed sutures. If this occurs take your sutures out and start again.

Late
- Infection/abscess formation.
- Bleeding (secondary haemorrhage).
- Wound breakdown.
- Skin necrosis.
- Suture displacement.
- Non-healing wound.
- Scarring.
- Loss of function.

Joint aspiration/arthrocentesis

Introduction
Joint aspiration (arthrocentesis) is a procedure of therapeutic and diagnostic importance for joint swellings. It must be performed in a competent, safe manner as it can potentially introduce infection into a previously sterile joint space.

Indications for joint aspiration
Therapeutic indications
- Drainage of a tense haemarthrosis <24 hours old.
- Drainage of a tense joint effusion for pain relief.

Diagnostic indications
- Evaluation of an unexplained arthritis with associated effusion.
- Clinical suspicion of a septic joint/crystal arthropathy.
- Evaluation of antibiotic sensitivities to a suspected septic joint.

Contraindications

- Overlying cellulitis.
- Coagulopathy.
- Thrombocytopenia.
- Prosthetic joint.

Brief anatomy of the knee joint

The knee joint is the largest and most commonly aspirated joint. A basic understanding of its anatomy is essential to perform a safe aspiration.

It is a synovial hinge joint with a wide range of movement. This range of movement is at the sacrifice of stability. The knee therefore has ligaments and menisci which act to improve the stability of the joint.

The main articulation is formed between the the condyles of the femur and tibia. This articulation is deepened by two c-shaped fibrocartilageous structures, menisci, which also absorb shock transmitted through the joint.

Four ligaments stabilise the knee joint.

- Anterior cruciate ligament (ACL), which prevents anterior displacement of the tibia on the femur.
- Posterior cruciate ligament (PCL), which prevents posterior displacement of the tibia on the femur.
- Medial and lateral collateral ligaments, which act to stabilise medial and lateral aspects of the knee joint, preventing separation of the femur from tibia (e.g. a blow to the lateral aspect of the knee joint will potentially strain the medial collateral ligament).

Joint capsule

The attachments of the joint capsule are complex but it is important to be aware of its anterior and lateral boundaries, as this will guide your placement of the needle during aspiration (Figure 21.6). The attachments are:

- medially – articular margin of the femur
- laterally – the groove of the popliteus tendon

- superiorly – superior to the patella it is continuous with the suprapatellar bursa – this bursa continues 5 cm superior to the patella normally
- inferiorly – attachments to the tibial condyles and both menisci

Step-by-step guide: knee aspiration lateral approach

- **Give a full explanation to the patient in simple terms and ensure they consent to the procedure.**
- **Set up your trolley (Box 21.2 and Figure 21.7).**
- **Prepare your trolley as a sterile field. Wear a plastic disposable apron and non-sterile gloves, and take alcohol hand rub with you.**

1 Place the patient relaxed in the supine position on a couch with a pillow under the knee, creating slight flexion of the joint.
2 Mark with a pen or surgical marker the point 1 cm superior and 1 cm lateral to the upper border of the patella.
3 Adopt universal precautions, set a sterile field, prepare the skin and drape the area (Figure 21.8a,b).
4 Anaesthetise the area around your aspiration site (Figure 21.8c).
5 With the brown cannula attached to a 20-mL syringe, advance through the previously marked spot at a direction 45° inferiorly and 45° down into the knee joint, attempting gentle aspiration as you advance.

Box 21.2 **Equipment for joint aspiration**

- Sterile pack, including drapes, a gallipot and gauze
- Sterile gloves
- Local anaesthetic
- 28G needle
- 5-mL syringe
- Brown intravenous cannula (14G venflon)
- 20-mL syringe
- Iodine-based solution for skin preparation (unless allergic)
- A minimum of two universal containers

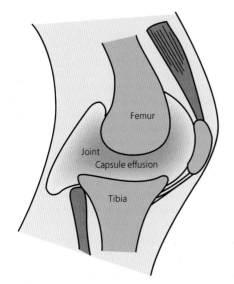

Figure 21.6 Knee joint.

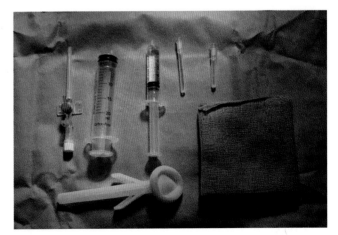

Figure 21.7 Equipment required for joint aspiration.

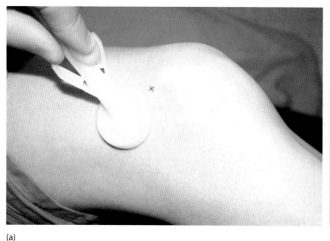

(a)

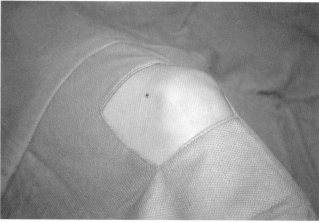

(b)

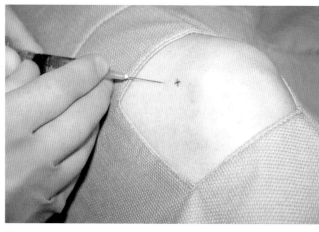

(c)

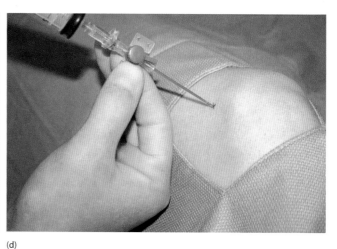

(d)

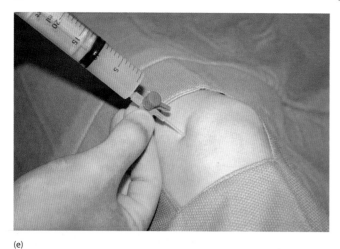

(e)

Figure 21.8 Step-by-step guide: joint (knee) aspiration. (a) Cleaning the marked knee. (b) Drape the area (a sterile field is of paramount importance in this procedure). (c) Infiltration of local anaesthetic. (d) Insertion of cannula into the joint space. (e) Aspiration of turbid fluid from knee joint.

6 As you enter the joint space you will feel a loss of resistance. At this point you will be able to aspirate joint contents (Figure 21.8d,e).

At this point you have the option of removing the needle from the cannula and aspirating through it directly using another 2-mL syringe. This will reduce the risk of iatrogenic trauma to the joint space lining and cartilage.

NB If aspiration is difficult, apply pressure on the medial aspect of the patella; this displaces fluid toward the lateral aspect of the patella.

The amount of fluid aspirated depends upon the aim of the procedure. Only a couple of millilitres of synovial fluid are required for analysis. If, however, you are performing the procedure for symptomatic relief you may continue aspirating until the patient is comfortable.

7 Once the aspiration is complete, withdraw the needle and apply pressure to the area with sterile gauze.

8 Place a sterile dressing over the site of aspiration.

9 Fully document the procedure, including consent, local anaesthetic and volume used, and colour and volume of the aspirate.

Samples to be sent

Place the aspirate into a minimum of two universal containers. These should be sent directly to the laboratory for crystal analysis, microscopy, Gram staining and culture.

Potential complications

Early

- Bleeding.
- Iatrogenic trauma to surrounding structures including the joint itself.
- Failed aspiration.
- Pain.

Late

- Infection/septic arthritis.
- Reaccumulation of joint fluid.

Handy hints/troubleshooting

- Remember to consider other options such as steristrip and gluing before you start – if in doubt ask advice from a senior.
- Make sure you have all your equipment ready before you start and that the area is well lit.
- Position yourself carefully – bending over awkwardly for half an hour isn`t going to help your back.
- Use plenty of local anaesthetic, antiseptic solution and irrigation.
- Take care to choose the appropriate size of suture.
- Nylon sutures can slip easily so use five knots for extra security.
- Don`t forget to check the patient`s tetanus status.

Further reading

Anderson LG. (1991) Aspirating and injecting the acutely painful joint. *Emerg Med* 23: 77–94.

Ma O, Cline D, Tintinalli J, Kelen G, Stapczynski J. (2004) *Emergency Medicine Just the Facts*, 2nd edn. McGraw-Hill, London.

Owen DS. (2004) Aspiration and injection of joints and soft tissues. In: Finestein G, Harris E, Budd R, McInnes I, Buddy S. (eds) *Kelly's Textbook of Rheumatology*, 7th edn. WB Saunders, Philadelphia.

Schumacher HR. (1997) Arthrocentesis of the knee. *Hosp Med* 33: 60–4.

Wyatt J, Illingworth R, Clancy M, Munro P, Robertson C. (2005) *Oxford Handbook of Accident and Emergency Medicine*, 2nd edn. Oxford University Press, Oxford.

CHAPTER 22

Specials: Paediatric Procedures

Kate McCann[1] and Amy Walker[2]

[1]*New Cross Hospital, Wolverhampton, UK*
[2]*Department of Neonatology, Birmingham Women's Hospital, Birmingham, UK*

OVERVIEW

By the end of this chapter you should be able to:

- understand the principles of performing practical procedures on children
- adequately prepare yourself, the environment, your equipment and the child for a procedure
- understand the indications and contraindications for various paediatric procedures
- describe how to perform a heel prick, take bloods, insert a cannula, perform a lumbar puncture, and perform a suprapubic urine aspiration on paediatric patients.

Box 22.1 **Preparing for paediatric procedures**

- Find an appropriate room.
- Decide on the tests required.
- Prepare appropriate equipment.
- Enlist holder and distracter.
- Wear protective gloves.
- Position yourself comfortably.
- Limit attempts to two or three.
- Have dressings, tape and sharps box within reach.

Introduction

It may be a cliché, but children are really not 'just small adults'. Several of the interventions described here are similar to the adult version, yet the approach requires more preparation. Though junior doctors may be proficient with adult procedures, children present a greater challenge and it is important not to become disheartened if it is initially a struggle. This chapter aims to provide useful tips and advice for completing common paediatric procedures.

Preparation

Preparation is the key to paediatric procedures (Box 22.1). Expect wriggling, screaming and both the child and parents becoming distressed. Verbal consent from parents must be gained for all procedures and should be documented.

Firstly, plan a suitable location. A simple heel prick can occur at the bedside, but more invasive tests should occur in neutral territory. Most wards will have a treatment room, since it is important for the child to consider their ward bed as a place of safety.

In advance, choose what equipment is needed and which tests are required. Inflicting pain in children should be minimised and blood tests anticipated, so that sampling is not unnecessarily repeated. Children's veins collapse at lower pressures so therefore we use gravity and venous pressure to collect blood. This requires preopening the bottles so that the blood can be dripped into them. Use a roll of tape to stand the filled bottles in, have preflushed tubing ready to connect to cannulae and adhesive dressings available to secure the line. Children will not stay still while you search for materials.

Holding the child securely and providing effective distraction will hugely improve the success of the procedure. Play therapists are specialised in distraction, but a family member or colleague can provide the required diversion. You may consider using dummies or sucrose (depending on local policy) to calm babies. Up until around 4 months, place babies in a cot or on a couch, with a colleague stabilising the limb. After this age, their strength requires a firm embrace (usually from a parent) along with limb stabilisation (see Figure 22.1). Older children may prefer to lie down, so always ask their preference.

Senior supervision is required for all procedures until you are competent to perform them alone. Limit your attempts to two or three for the benefit of both the child and the colleague who follows. When the task is over, ensure that cannulas are well secured with bandages and splints and allow parents to comfort the child.

Local anaesthetic creams

These are widely used in paediatrics. Unless the child is seriously unwell, apply anaesthetic cream before a painful procedure. Consult local hospital policy regarding age criteria for use.

Indications
- Cannulation, venepuncture and lumbar puncture.

Contraindications
- Previous adverse reaction, broken skin and severe eczema.
- EMLA® not recommended in neonates.

ABC of Practical Procedures. Edited by T. Nutbeam and R. Daniels. © 2010
Blackwell Publishing, ISBN: 978-1-4051-8595-0.

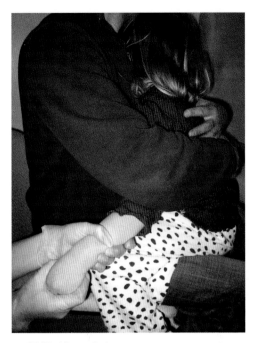

Figure 22.1 Child-holding technique.

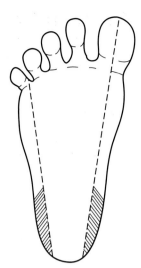

Figure 22.2 Shaded areas show where to perform heel prick.

Anatomy
- Examine first to identify veins.
- Put cream on multiple areas.

Procedure
- Apply layer of cream.
- Cover with occlusive dressing.
- Leave for 30–45 minutes (AMETOP®) or 1 hour (EMLA®).

Complications
- Skin reactions.
- Accidental ingestion.

Heel prick

This method for sampling small amounts of blood can be extremely useful for babies up to around 3 months of age.

Indications
- Blood sampling for capillary gases, basic biochemistry and full blood count.

Contraindications
- Not suitable for clotting, ammonia or blood cultures.
- Severe bruising, oedema or poor perfusion.

Anatomy
- Puncture heel in shaded areas as shown in Figure 22.2.

Procedure
- Wear protective gloves.
- Warm the foot before sampling.

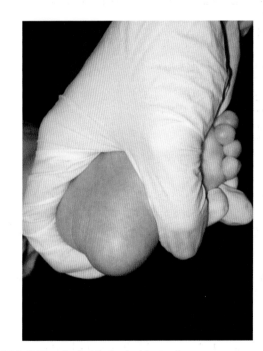

Figure 22.3 Holding the foot for heel prick sampling.

- Clean the area using a steret and apply a thin film of paraffin wax. This enables droplets of blood to form and makes collection easier.
- Hold the foot as shown in Figure 22.3 between fingers and thumb.
- Puncture the skin with an appropriate lancet. There are different-sized devices depending on the size of baby.
- Milk the blood down the foot held in dorsiflexion.
- Release the foot momentarily each time to ensure blood flows back into the foot.
- Avoid squeezing the foot – this often results in haemolysis and having to repeat the test.

Complications
- Infection and bruising.

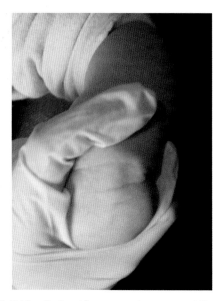

Figure 22.4 Holding the hand for venepuncture or cannulation.

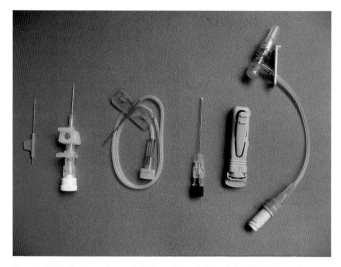

Figure 22.5 Commonly used devices. From left to right: blood sampling needle, Neoflon®, butterfly needle, lumbar puncture needle, heel prick device, T-piece to attach to cannulas.

Venepuncture

The general approach and skin preparation is the same as in Chapter 5.

Indications
- To obtain blood samples.

Contraindications
- None.

Anatomy
- For babies and toddlers – use dorsal surface of hands and feet.
- For older children – use the antecubital fossa.

Procedure
Hand or foot holding is crucial. With babies and small children, encircle the foot or hand with your own hand, whilst pulling the skin taut (Figure 22.4).
- For babies, use the blood-sampling needle (Figure 22.5). Insert slowly into a vein until blood drips from the end. Drip samples into bottles – mix coagulation and FBC bottles to avoid clotting.
- For toddlers, use a butterfly needle with the tubing removed. This creates a lower pressure in order to obtain samples.
- For older children, use a butterfly needle attached to a syringe. Don't pull back quickly on the syringe since the blood flows more slowly than in adults.

Complications
- Bruising.

Cannulation

Cannulation is indicated if a child requires intravenous fluids or antibiotics, but it is also reasonable to leave a cannula in after taking bloods if the decision to treat depends on the results.

Indications
- Intravenous medications and fluids.
- Frequent blood sampling (e.g. endocrine investigations).

Contraindications
- Avoid areas of broken skin (e.g. eczema).

Anatomy
- Veins that can be seen (less commonly palpated).
- Dorsum of hands and feet. Feet are often the first-line choice in babies and toddlers.
- Antecubital fossa or hands in older children. Avoid the antecubital fossa and long saphenous vein in neonates, as these are sites required for long lines.

Procedure
See Chapter 10 for a step-by-step guide to cannulation. Below is a list of helpful tips particular to paediatrics.
- Apply local anaesthetic.
- Preparation – see previous section.
- Cannula choice depends on the age of the child. For neonates and young infants use a Neoflon® (Figure 22.5). For toddlers and young children, where possible use a blue (22G) cannula. For older children and teenagers use a blue or pink cannula (20G).
- Avoid using a tourniquet except for older teenage patients.
- Hold the foot or hand as described above (Figure 22.4).
- Children's veins are very mobile. Be prepared to withdraw within the skin and try to pierce the vein again.
- Take it slowly – flashback is often slower due to the lower venous pressure.
- Apply tape over the 'nose' of the cannula when inserted.
- Drip blood into bottles.
- Connect a preflushed T-piece (Figure 22.5) to the cannula and flush. This can also be used to advance a cannula that is jammed against a valve.

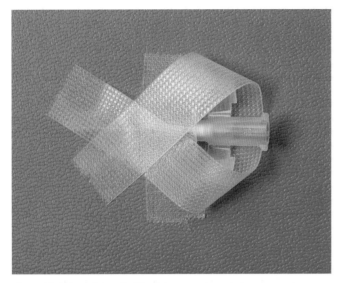

Figure 22.6 Butterfly method for fixing cannula.

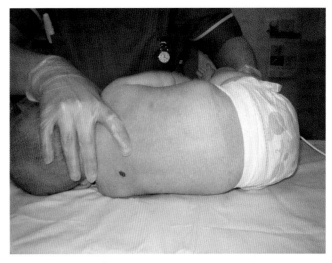

Figure 22.8 Positioning for lumbar puncture.

- Change the needle before inserting into the paediatric blood culture bottle.
- Alternatively, blood can be dripped into a 2-mL syringe with the plunger removed for blood cultures.

Lumbar puncture

The anatomical landmarks and general technique are as described in Chapter 7. The differences in children are related to size. Older children can be treated as adults but will need more reassurance and topical local anaesthetic. In younger children and babies, positioning and holding is the most important thing. Ensure that the person assisting you is familiar with the technique.

Indications
- Diagnosis of meningitis and metabolic investigation.

Contraindications
- Signs of raised intra-cranial pressure, focal neurological signs or clotting disorders.

Positioning (Figure 22.8)
- Place the child on an adjustable bed or cot at a comfortable height.
- Lie them on their side.
- Flex the shoulders and hips.
- Position the child with their back towards you on the edge of the surface.
- Keep the back straight in the vertical plane.

Procedure
- In all but larger children use the needle shown in Figure 22.5.
- Use aseptic technique as described in Chapters 3 and 7.
- Feel for the anterior superior iliac spine with your index finger and palpate for the intervertebral space perpendicular to this.

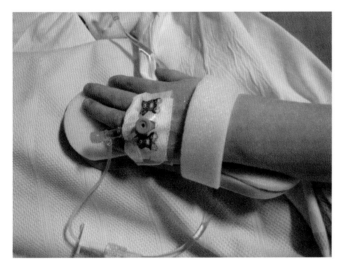

Figure 22.7 Splint device used for joint stabilisation.

- Fix securely – use the butterfly method with tape under the cannula flaps (Figure 22.6).
- Bandage well and use a splint to keep joints stable (Figure 22.7).

Complications
- Cellulitis, thrombophlebitis.
- It is not current practice to remove cannulas based on a specific time frame – the site should be monitored for signs of infection and removed accordingly.

Blood cultures from cannula

- Use a sterile green (21G) needle with a 2-mL syringe. Connecting the syringe directly can collapse the vein.
- Aspirate the blood (0.5–1 mL) from within the hub of the cannula. This method can also be used as an alternative to dripping blood into bottles.

- Insertion and collection is as described for adults in Chapter 7:
  - the needle will not need to be inserted as far as in adults
  - collect approximately 5–7 drops per container
  - use three universal containers for cell count, culture and protein with one glucose tube.
- Remove needle and cover site with plaster when finished.

Complications
- Bleeding (mild), infection (rare).
- Headache.

Suprapubic aspiration of urine

Indication
- To obtain an uncontaminated urine sample.

Contraindications
- Clotting disorders or thrombocytopenia.

Procedure
- Ideally confirm that there is urine in the bladder with ultrasound.
- Use aseptic technique.
- Attach a blue (23G) needle to a 5-mL syringe.
- Insert the needle into the abdomen 1 cm above the symphysis pubis perpendicular to the skin.
- Insert the needle to 2–3 cm, aspirating continuously until urine obtained.
- Remove needle and cover puncture site with a plaster.

Complications
- Bleeding.

An alternative sampling method is the in–out catheter. The technique is the same as for catheterisation except that the catheter is removed once a urine sample is obtained.

Blood gases

In paediatrics we rarely take arterial blood gases unless the patient has an arterial line. More commonly we rely on capillary or venous gases, collected via a capillary tube. This small glass tube is filled using heel or finger prick (capillary) or directly from venepuncture. The sample needs to be free flowing without any bubbles in the tube for accurate analysis (Figure 22.9).

Blood gases are interpreted in a similar manner to adults (see Chapter 6). Be mindful that some of the values will not be accurate. With venous gases, the pH and HCO_3 results are useful, but the reliability of the PCO_2 is debatable and should be interpreted with caution. Capillary gases are comparable with arterial gases for PCO_2, pH and HCO_3 but not PO_2. See Figure 22.10 for an introduction to analysing blood gases. Table 22.1 gives some causes of blood gases abnormalities.

Further procedures

There are several other procedures that would only be expected at a more senior level in paediatrics and neonatology. These include

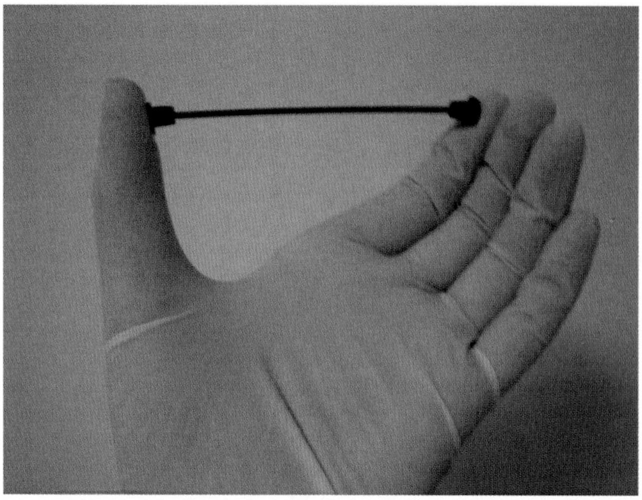

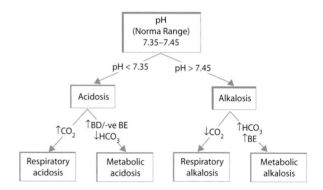

Figure 22.9 Filled capillary gas tube. Place bungs on either end and roll the tube between fingers to ensure mixing.

Figure 22.10 Analysis of blood gases. BD, base deficit; BE, base excess.

Table 22.1 Causes of blood gas abnormalities.

Respiratory acidosis
Poor respiratory drive
   (e.g. unconsciousness, neuromuscular disorders)
Respiratory diseases
   (e.g. asthma, bronchiolitis)

Metabolic acidosis
Diabetic ketoacidosis
Poor tissue perfusion
Renal disorders
   (e.g. renal tubular acidosis)
Inborn errors of metabolism
   (e.g. organic acidaemias)

Respiratory alkalosis
Hyperventilation
Salicylate poisoning (can also cause metabolic acidosis)

Metabolic alkalosis
Severe vomiting
   (e.g. pyloric stenosis)
Renal disorders
   (e.g. Bartter's syndrome)

long lines, umbilical catheters, intubation, chest drain and aspiration. The further reading list cites material that may be of use.

Handy hints/troubleshooting

Paediatric procedures are challenging yet fulfilling. Gaining the trust of the child is an important aspect of the process and a skill that will quickly develop with practice.
- Preparation is everything.
- Perform procedures in the appropriate place with enough assistance and equipment to hand.
- Always have senior supervision until full competence is achieved.
- Only perform necessary procedures (as infrequently as possible).
- Use appropriate techniques and support to minimise suffering.
- Always consult seniors when unsure.

Further reading

Lissauer T, Fanaroff A. (2006) *Neonatology at a Glance*. Blackwell Publishing Ltd, Oxford.

Mackway-Jones K, Molyneux E, Phillips B, Wieteska S. eds (2005) *Advanced Paediatric Life Support*, 4th edn. Blackwell Publishing, Oxford.

Silverman M, Henderson N, O'Callaghan C. (2009) *Practical Paediatric Procedures*. Hodder Arnold, London.

CHAPTER 23

Specials: Obstetrics and Gynaecology

Caroline Fox[1] and Lucy Higgins[2]

[1]*Birmingham Women's Hospital, Birmingham, UK*
[2]*Maternal and Fetal Health Research Centre, University of Manchester, St Mary's Hospital, Manchester, UK*

OVERVIEW

By the end of this chapter you should be able to:
- understand the indications and contraindications for insertion of vaginal speculum and bimanual examination
- be aware of the relevant anatomy for these procedures
- describe the procedure of performing vaginal speculum examination (with or without cervical smear)
- describe the procedure of performing bimanual examination.

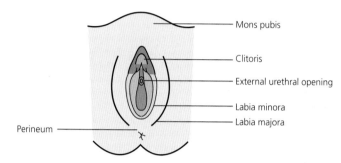

Figure 23.1 The vulva.

Vaginal speculum insertion with or without cervical smear

Indications
Allows visual inspection of the cervix and vaginal walls for the purposes of:
- diagnosing cervical/vaginal pathology (polyps, cancer, prolapse)
- detecting pre-invasive cervical disease (National Cervical Screening Programme)
- testing for lower genital tract infection including sexually transmitted infections (STIs)
- facilitating intrauterine instrumentation (e.g. IUCD, endometrial biopsy)
- investigating lower genital tract symptoms in pregnancy (e.g. bleeding, pain, discharge).

Contraindications
- Refusal of consent.
- Inability to take informed consent, unless to obtain information that will prevent harm or death.
- If the patient has never been sexually active they should be referred to a specialist. This also applies to paediatric patients.

Landmarks and anatomy
The female reproductive organs consist of the lower genital tract (vulva, vagina, cervix) and the upper genital tract (uterus, fallopian tubes and ovaries).

Vulva—Bounded by the mons pubis, labia majora and perineum. From anterior to posterior this contains the clitoris, external urethral opening, labia minora and vaginal introitus (external opening) – see Figure 23.1.

Vagina—A muscular tube extending superoposteriorly from the vaginal introitus to the uterus at the cervix. Superiorly the vagina is described in terms of anterior, posterior and lateral fornices. The superior aspect of the vagina is the widest part.

Cervix—Connects the uterine and vaginal cavities through the internal and external os. The endocervical canal is lined by mucus-secreting columnar epithelium whilst the vaginal surface is covered by squamous epithelium to resist the acidity of the vagina. The squamocolumnar junction (SCJ), is the area most susceptible to the malignant change of cervical cancer.

Uterus—A pear-shaped muscular organ.

Fallopian tubes—Arise from each cornu of the uterus and end at the ovaries.

Ovaries—Each ovary is oval and lies lateral to the uterus.

See Figure 23.2 – the female reproductive tract.

Equipment
- Disposable examination gloves.
- Cusco's bivalve speculum.

ABC of Practical Procedures. Edited by T. Nutbeam and R. Daniels. © 2010
Blackwell Publishing, ISBN: 978-1-4051-8595-0.

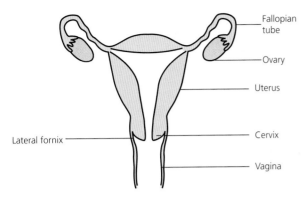

Figure 23.2 The female reproductive tract.

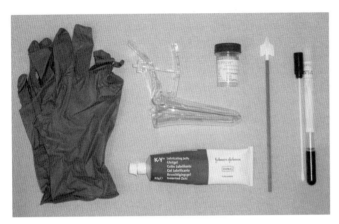

Figure 23.3 Equipment required to perform a speculum examination.

- Water-based lubricant.
- Cytobrush and vial of preservative solution.
- Sponge forceps and swab.
- Drape.
- Good light source.
- Suitable chaperone (preferably a trained observer but a friend/relative of the patient is acceptable if unavailable).

See Figure 23.3 for the equipment required to perform a speculum examination.

Step by guide: inserting a speculum

1 Firstly, check that the procedure is indicated; do you know what you are looking for?
2 Offer the patient a chaperone and document this in the notes. It is in your interest to have a chaperone present (obligatory for all male doctors).
3 Ensure that the environment is appropriate (private, adequate lighting etc.).
4 Explain why the procedure is necessary and what is going to happen, and gain informed consent. This intimate examination can make the patient feel vulnerable. Be mindful of this; act in a professional manner and treat the patient with respect and dignity. Ensure that your shirt sleeves, tie/scarf will not obstruct your examination. (Refer to your hospital policy regarding specific infection control policy regarding watches/short sleeves.)

5 Explain that slight discomfort is usual but reassure the patient that the test only takes a few minutes. Be aware of both verbal and non-verbal signs of distress or discomfort; if the patient wishes the examination to be stopped, this must be respected unequivocally.
6 The patient should undress from the waist downwards. Position the patient on the examination couch in a supine position. The patient bends her knees, places her heels together and lets her knees drop to either side (this is known as the lithotomy position). Adjust the light source so that it illuminates the vulva.
7 Most speculums are plastic and disposable, but if a metal speculum is used it may be warmed under running water. Apply lubricant to the blades of the speculum.
8 Hold the speculum with your dominant hand, with the opening mechanism pointing directly upwards and blades closed.
9 With your non-dominant hand, part the labia minora. Examine the vulva and labia for abnormalities (e.g. erythema, ulceration, warts and pigment changes).
10 Insert the speculum gently into the vagina; guide it towards the base of the spine with the blades at approximately 45° to the horizontal, adjusting the angle so the speculum passes with minimal resistance.
11 Once the speculum is fully inserted warn the patient that they will feel a stretching sensation and then slowly open the blades to visualise the cervix including the SCJ. By ensuring that the speculum is fully inserted you will open it at the vagina's widest point and minimise discomfort.
12 Next minimise expansion so that although the cervix is seen, the walls of the vagina are not stretched further than needed. Use the thumbscrew to hold the speculum open.
13 Inspect the cervix. If necessary remove excessive secretions using a swab. The epithelium should be uniformly pink. In some women (particularly those on oral contraceptives or in pregnancy) more columnar epithelium will be visible as a reddened area, known as an ectropion (a physiological change; erosion is an inaccurate term and describes ulceration, which would signify pathological change) (Figure 23.4).
14 Make note of any irregularity, friable tissue or ulceration.

To take a cervical smear

- Liquid-based cytology (LBC) is the current recommended method.
- Insert the brush into the cervix. Gently rotate through five full turns to sample the SCJ/TZ, maintaining good contact throughout.
- Remove the brush and detach its head or swill into the preservative solution (as per hospital policy).
- Label the vial with the patient's details.
- A small amount of bleeding after an examination is common so explain this to the patient; if there is excessive bleeding or you are concerned about the appearance of the cervix, further referral is necessary.

15 If you have concerns regarding STIs or abnormal vaginal discharge, microbiological swabs are indicated.

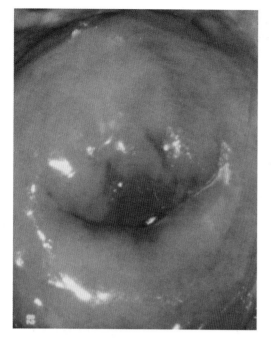

Figure 23.4 Cervix with small ectropion, the reddened area visible mainly on the upper lip of the cervix.

   ◦ Endocervical (two separate swabs: one chlamydia swab and a routine microbiology swab for gonorrhoea). Ensure two full turns of the swab against the endocervix before removal.
   ◦ Posterior fornix/high vaginal swab: routine microbiology swab. This is also the site for a fetal fibronectin test in threatened preterm labour.
16 To withdraw the speculum, loosen the thumbscrew but keep the blades slightly parted. This will prevent tissue being trapped and allow visualisation of the vaginal walls. Before removing the tip, close the blades completely.
17 If you suspect an STI, take a urethral swab for gonorrhoea and chlamydia.
18 A bimanual examination may be indicated; otherwise replace the drape, providing tissues and privacy for the patient.

Potential complications

A trained chaperone supports the patient, assists the practitioner and witnesses that all actions were necessary, appropriate and with consent. It is accepted practice that all doctors should conduct intimate examinations in the presence of a chaperone, by not doing so you expose yourself to unnecessary risk.

Handy hints/troubleshooting

- If visualisation of the cervical os is difficult you can withdraw the speculum slightly, ask the patient to place her fists at the base of her spine then reinsert the speculum and open the blades again. Alternatively, a longer speculum may be required.
- If applicable you can allow the patient's skirt to remain. This reduces exposure and perhaps anxiety.
- LBC enables a smear to be taken despite the presence of small amounts of blood; however, some women will be more comfortable being examined when they are not menstruating.

Specific requirements

For investigation of vaginal wall or uterine prolapse, a Simm's speculum allows better inspection of the vaginal walls. This is usually performed in the left lateral position.

Bimanual examination of the pelvis

Indications

- Evaluation of pelvic masses (fibroids, malignancy).
- Evaluation of pelvic pain (pelvic infection, endometriosis).

Contraindications

- As for speculum examination.
- Rarely performed in later stages of pregnancy, although a digital examination is useful to assess the cervix for diagnosis of labour.
- Any kind of digital examination is contraindicated in antepartum haemorrhage, until placenta praevia is excluded.
- Caution is necessary if an ectopic pregnancy is suspected, as too vigorous examination can cause rupture. If in doubt perform a speculum examination only.

Landmarks and anatomy

As for speculum examination. In addition, locate the anterior superior iliac spines and iliac crests.

Equipment

- Gloves.
- Lubricant gel.
- Drapes etc. as for speculum examination.

Step-by-step guide: bimanual examination of the pelvis

1 Firstly, check that the procedure is indicated; do you know what you are looking for?
2 Explain why the procedure is necessary, what will happen and gain informed consent. Perform abdominal palpation.
3 Explain that whilst slight discomfort is usual, the examination should not be painful and will last only a few minutes. Always perform abdominal palpation first.
4 The patient lies in the lithotomy position as for a speculum examination. Ensure that the abdomen is exposed for examination.
5 With the non-dominant hand, part the labia minora, again noting any visible lesions.
6 Lubricate the index and middle finger of the dominant hand and then insert through the vaginal introitus and rotate so that the finger pulps face superiorly.
7 Advance the examining fingers to the cervix.
   • Palpate the cervix for any irregularities. Note any pain on movement of the cervix (excitation).
   • Push the cervix superiorly, and place the non-dominant hand suprapubically gently pushing down to feel the uterus between both hands. Try to assess size and regularity of the uterus (a bulky irregular uterus suggests the presence of fibroids), mobility (immobility suggests adhesions from malignancy, pelvic infection, endometriosis or previous surgery). Note any tenderness.

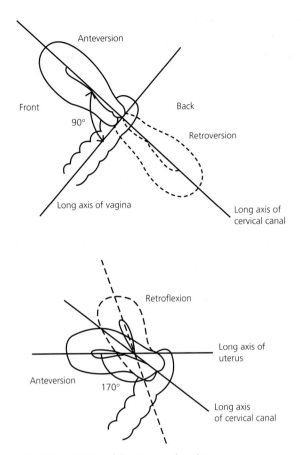

Figure 23.5 The positions of the uterus and cervix.

- Note whether the cervix is ante- or retroverted (angulated forward or backwards in relation to the vagina), and the uterus ante- or retroflexed (position in relation to the cervix).
  See Figure 23.5 for the positions of the uterus and cervix.
8 Pouch of Douglas.
- Continue gentle suprapubic pressure and move your fingers behind the cervix and feel for any nodules i.e. on the uterosacral ligaments from endometriosis.
9 Adnexae.
- Then move the non-dominant hand abdominally to approximately 4 cm medial from the iliac crest and your examining fingers vaginally into the right fornix to examine the right andexae. Gently sweep the abdominal hand downwards to palpate the adnexae between the two hands and assess size and tenderness. In the absence of any pathology the fallopian tubes and ovaries are often not palpable.
- Repeat on the opposite side, this time with the vaginal fingers in the left fornix.

10 Remove the examining fingers gently and inspect glove for blood/discharge.
11 Replace the drape over the woman's legs, providing tissues and privacy for the patient.

Potential complications
- As for speculum examination.

Specific requirements
- None

Handy hints/troubleshooting

- Start with the non-dominant hand high on the patient's abdomen to avoid missing substantial masses.
- An empty bladder makes palpation of the uterus easier.
- An acutely retroverted/retroflexed cervix/uterus may be difficult to palpate as may the uterus/ovaries in overweight or postmenopausal women.
- If the patient cannot relax the abdominal muscles to allow bimanual palpation, examination may be more successful carried out in the left lateral position.

Acknowledgements

We would like to thank Justin Clark for his help and guidance.

Further reading

National Institute for Health and Clinical Excellence. (2003) Liquid-based cytology for cervical screening. *NICE technology appraisal guidance 69.* www.nice.org.uk/nicemedia/pdf/TA69_LBC_review_FullGuidance.pdf

NHS Cervical Screening Programme. www.cancerscreening.nhs.uk/cervical/index.html

Royal College of General Practitioners: RCGP Sex, Drugs and HIV Task Group. *Sexually Transmitted Infections in Primary Care.* www.bashh.org/primarycare/stis_primary_care_march2006.pdf

Royal College of Obstetricians and Gynaecologists. *Clinical Governance Advice No. 6 (October 2004) Obtaining Valid Consent* www.rcog.org.uk/resources/Public/pdf/CGA_No6.pdf

Royal College of Obstetricians and Gynaecologists. *Gynaecological Examinations: Guidelines for Specialist Practice (July 2002)* www.rcog.org.uk/resources/public/pdf/WP_GynaeExams4.pdf)

Index

CURRENT TITLES

ABC of Skin Cancer

Edited by Sajjad Rajpar & Jerry Marsden
Sandwell & West Birmingham NHS Trust; Selly Oak Hospital, Birmingham

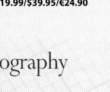

- A new, highly illustrated, concise, factual, and practical overview of skin cancers and pre-cancerous lesions
- Focuses on diagnosis, differential diagnosis, common pitfalls, and outlines best practice management in primary care
- In line with the latest NICE guidelines in the UK, places the emphasis on the pivotal role that GPs play in the screening, diagnosis and referral of skin cancers and pre-cancerous lesions
- Also includes chapters on non-surgical treatment and prevention

April 2008 | 9781405162197 | 80 pages | £19.99/$39.95/€24.90

ABC of Clinical Electrocardiography
SECOND EDITION

Edited by Francis Morris, William Brady & John Camm
Northern General Hospital, Sheffield; University of Virginia Health Sciences Centre, Charlottesville; St. George's University of London

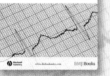

- A new edition of this practical guide to the interpretation of ECGs for the non-specialist
- The *ABC* format lends itself to clearly illustrate full 12-lead ECGs
- Sets out the main patterns seen in cardiac disorders in clinical practice, covering the fundamentals of interpretation and analysis
- Covers exercise tolerance testing and provides clear anatomical illustrations to explain key points

May 2008 | 9781405170642 | 112 pages | £26.99/$49.95/€34.90

ABC of Complementary Medicine
SECOND EDITION

Edited by Catherine Zollman, Andrew J. Vickers & Janet Richardson
General Practitioner, Bristol; Memorial Sloan-Kettering Cancer Center, New York; University of Plymouth

- This thoroughly revised and updated second edition offers an authoritative introduction to complementary therapies
- Includes the latest information on efficacy of treatments
- Places a new emphasis in patient management
- Ideal guide for primary care practitioners

June 2008 | 9781405136570 | 64 pages | £21.99/$40.95/€27.90

ABC of Eating Disorders

Edited by Jane Morris
Royal Edinburgh Hospital

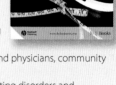

- Charts the diagnosis of different eating disorders and their management and treatment by GPs, dieticians and psychiatrists
- Examines diagnosis, management and treatment by health professionals and through self-help
- Helps primary care practitioners recognise eating disorders in young people presenting with other problems
- Supports the work of general psychiatrists and physicians, community health teams and teaching staff
- Includes medico-legal aspects of treating eating disorders and specialist referral

August 2008 | 9780727918437 | 80 pages | £19.99/$35.95/€24.90

ABC of Tubes, Drains, Lines and Frames

Edited by Adam Brooks, Peter F. Mahoney & Brian Rowlands
Queen's Medical Centre, University of Nottingham; The Royal Centre for Defence Medicine; The Royal Centre for Defence Medicine

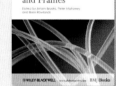

- A brand new title in the *ABC* series
- A full-colour, practical guide to the key issues involved in the assessment and management of surgical adjuncts
- Covers the care of post-operative patients in primary care
- Highlights common pitfalls and includes "trouble shooting" sections

October 2008 | 9781405160148 | 88 pages | £19.99/$35.95/€24.90

ABC of Headache

Edited by Anne MacGregor & Alison Frith
Both The City of London Migraine Clinic

- Uses real case histories to guide the reader through symptoms to diagnosis and management or, where relevant, to specialist referral
- A highly illustrated, informative and practical source of knowledge and offers links to further information and resources
- An essential guide for healthcare professionals, at all levels of training, looking for possible causes of presenting symptoms of headache

October 2008 | 9781405170666 | 88 pages | £19.99/$35.95/€24.90

For more information on any of the titles, please visit the *ABC* website at **www.abcbookseries.com**

ALSO AVAILABLE

ABC of Adolescence
Russell Viner
2005 | 9780727915740 | 56 pages | £19.99/$35.95/€24.90

ABC of Aids, 5th Edition
Michael W. Adler
2001 | 9780727915030 | 128 pages | £24.99/$46.95/€32.90

ABC of Alcohol, 4th Edition
Alexander Paton & Robin Touquet
2005 | 9780727918147 | 72 pages | £19.99/$35.95/€24.90

ABC of Allergies
Stephen R. Durham
1998 | 9780727912367 | 65 pages | £24.99/$44.95/€32.90

ABC of Antenatal Care, 4th Edition
Geoffrey Chamberlain & Margery Morgan
2002 | 9780727916921 | 92 pages | £22.99/$41.95/€29.90

ABC of Antithrombotic Therapy
Gregory Y.H. Lip & Andrew D. Blann
2003 | 9780727917713 | 67 pages | £19.99/$35.95/€24.90

ABC of Asthma, 5th Edition
John Rees & Dipak Kanabar
2005 | 9780727918604 | 80 pages | £24.99/$44.95/€32.90

ABC of Brainstem Death, 2nd Edition
Christopher Pallis & D.H. Harley
1996 | 9780727902450 | 55 pages | £25.99/$46.95/€32.90

ABC of Breast Diseases, 3rd Edition
J. Michael Dixon
2005 | 9780727918284 | 120 pages | £27.99/$50.95/€34.90

ABC of Burns
Shehan Hettiaratchy, Remo Papini & Peter Dziewulski
2004 | 9780727917874 | 56 pages | £19.99/$35.95/€24.90

ABC of Child Protection, 4th Edition
Sir Roy Meadow, Jacqueline Mok & Donna Rosenberg
2007 | 9780727918178 | 120 pages | £27.99/$50.95/€34.90

ABC of Clinical Genetics, 3rd Edition
Helen M. Kingston
2002 | 9780727916273 | 120 pages | £25.99/$47.95/€32.90

ABC of Clinical Haematology, 3rd Edition
Drew Provan
2007 | 9781405153539 | 112 pages | £27.99/$50.95/€34.90

ABC of Colorectal Cancer
David Kerr, Annie Young & Richard Hobbs
2001 | 9780727915269 | 39 pages | £19.99/$35.95/€24.90

ABC of Colorectal Diseases, 2nd Edition
David Jones
1998 | 9780727911056 | 110 pages | £27.99/$50.95/€34.90

ABC of Conflict and Disaster
Anthony Redmond, Peter F. Mahoney, James Ryan, Cara Macnab & Lord David Owen
2005 | 9780727917263 | 80 pages | £19.99/$35.95/€24.90

ABC of COPD
Graeme P. Currie
2006 | 9781405147118 | 48 pages | £19.99/$35.95/€24.90

ABC of Diabetes, 5th Edition
Peter J. Watkins
2002 | 9780727916938 | 108 pages | £27.99/$50.95/€34.90

ABC of Ear, Nose and Throat, 5th Edition
Harold S. Ludman & Patrick Bradley
2007 | 9781405136563 | 120 pages | £27.99/$50.95/€34.90

ABC of Emergency Radiology, 2nd Edition
Otto Chan
2007 | 9780727915283 | 144 pages | £29.99/$53.95/€37.90

ABC of Eyes, 4th Edition
Peng T. Khaw, Peter Shah & Andrew R. Elkington
2004 | 9780727916594 | 104 pages | £25.99/$46.95/€32.90

ABC of Health Informatics
Frank Sullivan & Jeremy Wyatt
2006 | 9780727918505 | 56 pages | £19.99/$35.95/€24.90

ABC of Heart Failure, 2nd Edition
Russell C. Davis, Michael K. Davies & Gregory Y.H. Lip
2006 | 9780727916440 | 72 pages | £19.99/$35.95/€24.90

ABC of Hypertension, 5th Edition
Gareth Beevers, Gregory Y.H. Lip & Eoin O'Brien
2007 | 9781405130615 | 88 pages | £24.99/$44.95/€32.90

ABC of Intensive Care
Mervyn Singer & Ian Grant
1999 | 9780727914361 | 64 pages | £17.99/$31.95/€24.90

ABC of Interventional Cardiology
Ever D. Grech
2003 | 9780727915467 | 51 pages | £19.99/$35.95/€24.90

ABC of Kidney Disease
David Goldsmith, Satishkumar Abeythunge Jayawardene & Penny Ackland
2007 | 9781405136754 | 96 pages | £26.99/$49.95/€34.90

ABC of Labour Care
Geoffrey Chamberlain, Philip Steer & Luke Zander
1999 | 9780727914156 | 60 pages | £18.99/$33.95/€24.90

ABC of Learning and Teaching in Medicine
Peter Cantillon, Linda Hutchinson & Diana Wood
2003 | 9780727916785 | 64 pages | £18.99/$33.95/€24.90

ABC of Liver, Pancreas and Gall Bladder
Ian Beckingham
2001 | 9780727915313 | 64 pages | £18.99/$33.95/€24.90

ABC of Major Trauma, 3rd Edition
Peter Driscoll, David Skinner & Richard Earlam
1999 | 9780727913784 | 192 pages | £24.99/$46.95/€32.90

ABC of Mental Health
Teifion Davies & T.K.J. Craig
1998 | 9780727912206 | 120 pages | £27.99/$50.95/€34.90

ABC of Monitoring Drug Therapy
Jeffrey Aronson, M. Hardman & D. J. M. Reynolds
1993 | 9780727907912 | 46 pages | £19.99/$35.95/€24.90

ABC of Nutrition, 4th Edition
A. Stewart Truswell
2003 | 9780727916648 | 152 pages | £25.99/$46.95/€32.90

ABC of Obesity
Naveed Sattar & Mike Lean
2007 | 9781405136747 | 64 pages | £19.99/$33.95/€24.90

ABC of Occupational and Environmental Medicine, 2nd Edition
David Snashall & Dipti Patel
2003 | 9780727916112 | 124 pages | £27.99/$50.95/€34.90

ABC of One To Seven, 4th Edition
Bernard Valman
1999 | 9780727912329 | 156 pages | £27.99/$50.95/€34.90

ABC of Oral Health
Crispian Scully
2000 | 9780727915511 | 41 pages | £18.99/$33.95/€24.90

ABC of Palliative Care, 2nd Edition
Marie Fallon & Geoffrey Hanks
2006 | 9781405130790 | 96 pages | £23.99/$44.95/€29.90

ABC of Patient Safety
John Sandars & Gary Cook
2007 | 9781405156929 | 64 pages | £22.99/$40.95/€29.90

ABC of Preterm Birth
William McGuire & Peter Fowlie
2005 | 9780727917638 | 56 pages | £19.99/$35.95/€24.90

ABC of Psychological Medicine
Richard Mayou, Michael Sharpe & Alan Carson
2003 | 9780727915566 | 72 pages | £19.99/$35.95/€24.90

ABC of Resuscitation, 5th Edition
Michael Colquhoun, Anthony Handley & T.R. Evans
2003 | 9780727916693 | 111 pages | £27.99/$50.95/€34.90

ABC of Rheumatology, 3rd Edition
Michael L. Snaith
2004 | 9780727916884 | 136 pages | £25.99/$46.95/€32.90

ABC of Sexual Health, 2nd Edition
John Tomlinson
2004 | 9780727917591 | 96 pages | £24.99/$44.95/€32.90

ABC of Sexually Transmitted Infections, 5th Edition
Michael W. Adler, Frances Cowan, Patrick French, Helen Mitchell & John Richens
2004 | 9780727917614 | 104 pages | £24.99/$46.95/€32.90

ABC of Smoking Cessation
John Britton
2004 | 9780727918185 | 56 pages | £17.99/$33.95/€22.90

ABC of Sports and Exercise Medicine, 3rd Edition
Gregory Whyte, Mark Harries & Clyde Williams
2005 | 9780727918130 | 136 pages | £27.99/$53.95/€34.90

ABC of Subfertility
Peter Braude & Alison Taylor
2004 | 9780727915344 | 64 pages | £18.99/$33.95/€24.90

ABC of the Upper Gastrointestinal Tract
Robert Logan, Adam Harris, J.J. Misiewicz & J.H. Baron
2002 | 9780727912664 | 54 pages | £19.99/$35.95/€24.90

ABC of Urology, 2nd Edition
Chris Dawson & Hugh N. Whitfield
2006 | 9781405139595 | 64 pages | £21.99/$40.95/€27.90

ABC of Wound Healing
Joseph E. Grey & Keith G. Harding
2006 | 9780727916952 | 56 pages | £19.99/$35.95/€24.90